The Psyche of the Body

T0231411

The Psyche of the Body is a passionate and well-informed plea for a Jungian version of psychosomatic medicine and psychotherapy. Many cases of physical illness show evidence of the effect of psychic involvement, both in origin and treatment. Yet to date, the majority of study into psychosomatic illness has been purely empirical, with little theory to help interpret and put results into context.

Illustrated by vivid clinical illustrations of case histories, *The Psyche of the Body* reviews the long history of psychosomatic medicine and models of the relationship between psyche and body that have evolved over time, and presents a full revision of research in the field over the last twenty years. It presents a much-needed theoretical model together with practical guidelines that demonstrate how the psychological aspects of specific illnesses should be handled in therapy and analysis.

Practicing and training Jungian analysts, as well as all those involved in clinical treatment, will find the interdisciplinary approach to psychosomatic medicine promoted in this book fascinating reading.

Denise Gimenez Ramos is a clinical psychologist and member of the Brazilian Society of Analytical Psychology. She has a private clinic in São Paulo and is Professor of Analytical Psychology and Head of the Department of Post-Graduate Studies in Clinical Psychology at the Pontifícia Universidade Católica de São Paulo. She is also Chair of the Academic Sub-Committee and Vice-President of the International Association for Analytical Psychology.

The Psyche of the Body

A Jungian approach to psychosomatics

Denise Gimenez Ramos

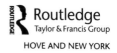
Routledge
Taylor & Francis Group

HOVE AND NEW YORK

First published in Portuguese as *A Psique do Corpo*
by Summus Editorial, São Paulo, Brazil

First published in English 2004
by Routledge
27 Church Road, Hove, East Sussex BN3 2FA

Simultaneously published in the USA and Canada
by Routledge
711 Third Avenue, New York, NY 10017

Routledge is an imprint of the Taylor&Francis Group

Copyright © 2004 Denise Gimenez Ramos

Typeset in Great Britain by RefineCatch Limited, Bungay, Suffolk

Paperback cover design by Hybert Design
Paperback cover illustration "Does the Onion Man Cry?"
by Paulo Gruber

British Library Cataloguing in Publication Data
A catalogue record for this book is available from the British Library

Library of Congress Cataloging-in-Publication Data
Ramos, Denise Gimenez, 1947–
 [Psique do corpo. English]
 The psyche of the body: 'a Jungian approach to psychosomatics' /
Denise Gimenez Ramos.
  p. cm.
 Includes bibliographical references and index.
 ISBN 1-58391-897-3 (alk. paper)—ISBN 1-58391-898-1
(pbk.: alk. paper)
 1. Medicine, Psychosomatic. 2. Jungian psychology.
3. Psychotherapy. 4. Mind and body. 5. Diseases—Philosophy.
I. Title.
  RC49.R266 2004
  616'.0019–dc22   2004003890

ISBN13: 978–1–583–91897–5 (hardback)
ISBN13: 978–1–583–91898–2 (paperback)

In memory of:

Maria da Penha Gimenez
Nilo Ramos
René Victor Liviano

They have left us with the great mystery and with the desire to get it right more and more each time.

Contents

Figures

Acknowledgments

So many were my teachers over the course of these years that it would be impossible to cite them all here by name. I should, however, mention those who have played the most direct role in developing the present work: Lúcia B. Kohler and Luiz C. Figueiredo, who contributed to my work with their valuable suggestions and guidance, and Liliana L. Wahba for the inspiring words, thoughts and support that only a true friend could give.

I should especially like to thank Dr Mathilde Neder. I regard it as a privilege to have had the guidance of Dr Neder, pioneer and teacher who, above all through her example, brought a sense of worthiness to each step and to each discovery. Her enthusiasm and affection were present throughout.

I thank Paul Brutsche and the Susan Bach Foundation for the grant that allowed me to translate this book, and to Andrew Samuels for his friendship and support.

To my patients, I send my gratitude for the trust they deposited in me, to which I hope to do justice and respect with humility. To my students, who, with their intriguing questions, caused me to rethink what I had known for certain. To Pericles Machado for his valuable assistance with the revision of the last researches, papers and data. To Robin Geld and Lincoln Berkley for assistance with the translation.

And finally, to Viviane, who, in the wisdom of her eight years (on the occasion of my doctorate), coming upon her mother submerged under masses of papers, sent me a note:

Yet a passion.
The science of the thesis is to show that a person may transform one thing into
Something else, however . . .

At the time, she said she didn't know how it should finish, and now, 10 years later, I must confess that the increase of the complexity of our knowledge convinces me that there is not really an end for these fascinating questions.

Introduction

We cannot rid ourselves of the doubt that perhaps this whole separation of mind and body may finally prove to be merely a device of reason for the purpose of conscious discrimination – an intellectually necessary separation of one and the same fact into two aspects, to which we then illegitimately attribute an independent existence.

(Jung, 1972: 619)

Not long ago, I was surprised by a phone call from the intensive care unit of a hospital. In a voice that seemed very anxious, an ex-patient of mine asked, "How did you guess that I would have a heart attack, when all my clinical exams were normal? My doctor himself told me that I was in fine shape and two months later, I have a heart attack!"

As it was not the right moment for great explanations, we talked about what had happened and set a time for my visit to the hospital. But I spent quite some time thinking about how I would explain to the patient that I had not guessed what was to happen and that my asking him to take care of his health had not been an intuitive flash. Rather, my recommendation had been based on a theoretical model backed by research that allowed me to predict such a happening with a certain margin of confidence.

This example, among so many others in clinical practice and our daily meetings, reveals clearly the obtuseness that still prevails among a high number of professionals in the health field. Although this patient had been complaining for quite some time about love and "cardiac" pains, as these were not detected by the state of the art in technology, they went by unheeded by the cardiologist. However, the patient's dreams, his complexes, his hasty behavior, his contained anger and hostile attitude towards all who did not follow his orders at once, were visible factors of a heart risk. Not getting any feedback from the doctor, the patient gave up analysis, finding his afflictions to be "nothing that a vacation could not solve" (doctor's words). The patient had a heart attack on the beach, on his second day of vacation. What was it that happened, he wanted to know. What happened was the traditional split between the living, subjective body and the body of biology, the body of anatomy and physiology classes. The patient was a victim of the Cartesian body/spirit/psyche division. He almost died from "this".

Unconsciously, we perpetuate a vision wherein detailed, minute descriptions derived from dissections or physiological studies prevail over the perception of feelings and the subjective and symbolic sensations of the body.

In this discrepancy between the described body and the living body lies one of the central difficulties in arriving at a common language between medicine and psychology. Having for so many years been dissociated, these two fields of knowledge suffer from mutual prejudices that hinder both. Even psychosomatics – the youngest daughter of this wedding – suffers from the same neurosis in trying to reduce pathologies to a cause-and-effect psychology, using the reductionist biomedical method.

Thus, frustrated with the dearth of theoretical and method-ological research attempting to determine a relation between psycho-logical and physiological phenomena, in my PhD thesis in 1993 I established a theoretical field that allowed a broader, more scientific basis in the area.

At the time, the word "psychosomatics" had already been exe-crated by many scientists for being remindful in some way of the psychologism of the 1970s, which resulted in the patients' being held responsible for their pains and sufferings. Thus, besides worrying about their illnesses, patients were made to blame for their sadness, not dealing adequately with their mourning, having such and such personality traits, or for being chronic depressives. At the same time, the efficacy of surgery and medication stood up against vague psy-chological notions such as "death wish", "lack of enthusiasm for life", among others. Psychological theories also contributed little to the understanding of the psyche–body phenomenon, in that they either remained at a superficial, behavioral level or reduced the phe-nomenon psychodynamically to traumatic child causes, with few efficient therapeutic resources.

This problem is still reflected in the most diverse of present-day circumstances. It is evident in the two schools of medicine and psychology, which fight over the human being, each one sticking to its truth and side and, worse still, thinking its side to be the totality. This pretentious inflation, among other consequences, has resulted in considerable scientific setbacks and a debilitating one-sidedness in science and consciousness.

At the same time, patients, afflicted by their symptoms, divide themselves into pieces, revealing each one of these to different professionals, who frequently reinforce the "schizophrenization" of the patients, when not provoking it themselves. Both doctor and patient, as part of their cultural context, have little awareness of this process, thinking the different directions quite correct. Moreover, it is generally the case where "organic causes" have been excluded that attention is directed to psychology, which is responsible only for "emotionally disturbed" patients, once again reinforcing the "schizophrenia" prevalent within our professional circles.

The recent coining of terms such as "psychocardiology", "psychooncology", "psychoneuroimmunology" and "psychoendocrinology" so as to avoid "psychosomatics", while serving to delimitate an area of studies, also continues to reflect the dichotomy of the body and goes against the grain of history, as increasingly the interrelation between various systems is revealed. It is not possible to speak of psychocardiology without studying psychoendocrinology, for instance.

This problem can be understood as the result of an evolutionary process. We are determined by the myths and beliefs of our times; thus, understanding these is essential in bringing to light what has determined our attitudes regarding health and disease (Chapter 2).

Today we are seeing an enormous advance, especially in the field of neuroscience: a promising source for understanding the relations between the nervous system, brain and mind. Alongside this, there is an accumulation in psychology of a vast set of experiments which, while highly polemic, have been confirming the influence of psychosocial variables on the origin and development of so-called organic diseases (I say here "so-called organic" for lack of better terminology, in that I consider all diseases, physical and mental, psycho-organic).

However, in Chapter 5 we will see that the development of most of the studies in this field has been purely empirical, with little or generally no theory to give them substance. In most of the studies there is proof of psychic involvement both in the origin and in the treatment of organic illnesses. The lack of depth of the theories, together with the poor theoretical body, has created great difficulty in the interpretation of the results, which are limited to the variables studied.

The psychological theories in general, when applied to these areas, have used for the most part a classical, deterministic, mechanical methodology, no longer in keeping with the new scientific models. Even worse, they do not allow for the understanding of phenomena that escape the narrow lens that such methodology imposes. There is an urgent need for the development of a coherent theoretical body, which can more widely encompass the vastness of a theme as complex as the question of the psyche–body phenomenon in illnesses. Support for this proposal is to be found in analytical psychology, and it is with this question in mind that this study is developed (Chapters 3 and 4).[1]

This book is an updated edition of the original, published in Portuguese in 1994. It was written primarily for healthcare students and professionals, many of whom are not familiar with Jungian terminology, aiming to develop a theoretical psychological model to be applied in the understanding and treatment of organic diseases within modern scientific standards.

In the 10 years following the original edition, much research has given continuity to this work, including a great deal of postgraduate clinical psychology research. The model developed has also been used by psychologists and doctors in hospital care, and has proved highly promising in the investigation of cardiovascular diseases and cancer in particular. Recently, it was also applied in the study of patients with lupus, vitiligo, heart diseases and terminal diseases, with excellent results.

In Chapter 6 we will examine three cases of organic illnesses in psychotherapy, followed by other vignettes (Chapter 7). The objectives are: (1) to understand the illnesses in light of the developed analytical model and compare them to the data produced by the research; and (2) using the analytical model and its psychotherapeutic techniques, to observe the changes in the patients' organic symptoms.

We will see that the use of the analytical model in patients with organic symptoms leads to an improvement in their general health and at the same time heightens their level of consciousness. Even when there is no organic improvement due to the irreversibility of the clinical state, it is evident that the patient, in understanding the process and being able to attribute to it a symbolic meaning, feels relief and a greater sense of well-being.

Chapter 1

Some models and concepts of disease and the healing process

The emerging paradigm brings to the surface of our consciousness, in a more detailed scientific form, what we, and our fathers and forefathers before us, have known all along.

(Laszlo, 1993: 223)

There are many myths and models today that determine how we view health and sickness and deal with them. They originate with the history of humans and evolve in tandem with the evolution of human consciousness. They are present simultaneously and paradoxically.

Humans in the information technology era appeal to the gods on the moment of pain, in search of the meaning of their suffering. However developed society may be, the mystery of life and death remains. Reason and faith, scientific and religious concepts are mixed in modern people who search for meaning, and determine their attitude in the face of health and sickness.

Myths mold our perception of the world and of the phenomena that we propose to study. They were created in the search for the meaning of life, and through them we come to have a more rational understanding of the world that surrounds us. According to the great scientist Joseph Campbell:

Myths are the metaphors of the human beings' spiritual potential. They relate us to nature and with the natural world.

(Campbell, 1990: 6)

The practice of the science of healing always reflects the morals, the ethics, the myths, and the psychological development of the culture of which it is a part. In the following pages we shall briefly discuss some of these myths and models, especially those that are still with us today.

To broaden our perspective, we can observe the development of the understanding of the process of sickness and healing as an example of the collective process of individuation, from the psychological point of view, as described by C.G. Jung. This allows a meta-analysis and a more discriminating understanding of the models that determine our clinical and research attitudes.

According to the analytical model, the ego, at birth, is immersed in the totality of the Self without discrimination between the I and the non-I. The pre-egoic state is a paradisiacal, unitary, non-divided state. The appearance of consciousness comes from the rupture of this indiscriminate totality. Slowly, certain contents of the unconscious start to separate and form the consciousness, this process being described by M. Fordham as "de-integration" (Fordham, 1957). What used to be a whole, One, becomes many. The original psychic structures have to be constantly broken, divided, to be integrated into the consciousness.

We shall see that the models collectively suffer the same process, and at the start of this century, after many "de-integrations", we are arriving at a moment where a new mandala becomes complete, closing a long circuit of "integrateds".

The primitive model

We have observed that the original unity is found to be much more preserved in children and in primitive people than in modern humans. In the latter, the superimposing of conscious structures aggregated around the ego has caused them to draw apart from their source, from their Self.

In primitive peoples, we see humans subjugated by the power of the forces of nature that their mind cannot understand. Humans equated these with divine powers, thus finding a temporary answer to their anguish in face of the unpredictable. Matter contained life, and natural events were personalized. Humans and nature were One.

Jung used the Levy-Bruhl's designation for this process, "participation mystique", which "denotes a peculiar kind of connection with object and consists in the fact that the subject cannot clearly distinguish himself from the object": "This identity results from an a priori oneness of subject and object" between ego and Self (Jung, 1971: 781). We find this original unity as source of life and of consciousness in very different myths on creation and cosmic events. Reality that explained life was invisible and non-material. A "spirit of totality" integrated all the elements of existence.

If, for primitive peoples, life had to be lived in accordance with the natural order of the spirit, it was a natural consequence that their therapeutic procedures would have the same focus (Mauceri, 1986).

The quality of observing nature as transcendent is found in the majority of archaic religions and led to the development of medicine, where respect for the spiritual and for the search for greater significance as regards disease and health were basic. The one who cured was the mediator between cosmic forces and the patient, and his value was based on the belief that he was an extension of the relationship of the primitive with the cosmos.

The shaman was the specialist who mediated this order to the patient. Myths were transmitted by word and materialized in totems and in images. The shaman, as mediator, had, therefore, the function of contacting spiritual forces. A cure was never attributed to him. His status was earned through his ability to precipitate "ecstasy". He would listen to the patient's history not in search of a symptom, but rather to discover what the patient's error had been. The disease was invariably the outcome of violating a taboo or offense to the gods. A cure lay in re-establishing the link of the human with the divine through repentance and sacrifice.

This idea also appears in the Bible, where we might consider Miriam, the first recorded example of punitive disease in Jewish–Christian culture. On criticizing her brother Moses for marrying an Ethiopian woman (dark skin), Miriam's own skin "became sickly and white as snow" (leprosy) and was cured only after seven days of repentance and sacrifice (Numbers 12:1–15).

Rituals of different types, offers to placate the divine wrath, and techniques for sacrifice were developed. One good example is found amid the Tucano Indians in the Amazon region, where disease is known as *doré*, a term derived from *doréri*, which signifies "that which was sent, to order". Disease among these Indians is interpreted as a product sent by a supernatural agent, as a form of punishment to those who disobey the moral norms of the tribe. On the other hand, *doréri* also means "to transform into something by means of the imagination" and, in this sense, disease and transformation are interconnected concepts. Here disease may have many causes (different transgressions) but always a purpose: "transformation".

The supernatural agent who has "sent" the disease, usually in the form of an animal, must be discovered and transformed, just as the patient is transformed when he interacts in his imagination with this animal, until he has subdued the animal. The function of the shaman is to intermediate this discovery by "invoking" invisible powers and strengthening the body by means of infusions and beverages (Reichel-Dolmatoff, 1971).

Thus, as the primitive medicine man also had knowledge of the medicinal properties of herbs, of music, and of verbal therapy (words were of great power in a non-literate culture), he provided two basic necessities of humans: a spiritual search and health.

All the civilizations that succeeded primitive society lent continuity to this train of thought. The Hindu, Egyptian, Chinese, Babylonian, Chaldean, Persian and ancient Greek civilizations built cosmogenic myths and had astronomy and "cure" as basic "science". In all these cultures, we can perceive the interconnection between empirical ability and spiritual belief (Solié, 1976).

The medicine man–doctor–priest fulfilled the physical and spiritual needs of the patient in such a way as to conserve the harmony between psyche and nature. To a certain extent, the shaman was a forerunner of the use of the techniques of trance, psychodrama, dream analysis, suggestion, and imagination. However, while the shaman remembers the values of his culture with his patient, through collective myths, the modern psychotherapist seeks the patient's personal myth in his unconscious past.

Perhaps one of the great differences between primitive and modern humans is precisely this excessive "personalism". In an era of rationalism and technical knowledge, humans can dissociate from religious values and those of nature. The religious need became dissociated from the culture. Modern humans began to believe that through science and technology they might prevail over nature and that, therefore, the need for the spiritual, for significance, would be less relevant. And this has been one of the myths of our era, inherited from Greek medicine – the most important and perhaps the most developed science among the Greek people.

The Greek model

The Greek physicians were the first to separate the spiritual category from the material, and to develop a scientific approach such as we use today: observation, analysis, deduction, and synthesis.

Separating the study of beings and of the qualities of spiritual life was a prerequisite in order for Greek philosophers to understand natural phenomena. However, the idea of a controlling principle in the cosmos remained indispensable as a first reality in cosmology. The concept of *Nous*, director intelligence, was considered the creative force that differentiated the material world through its ordinating activity. *Nous* was not on a par with a personal creator, God; it was closer to the idea of God, the Creator. To the Greek doctors, the world and the cosmos were recognizable and order prevailed in the multiplicity of things and in the unity of mutable diversity.

Use of music and the words of a spell were in common use in processes of cure. All acknowledged the curing power ("magic") of the words and used them to expel "daimons", the malevolent spirits of disease. Internal harmony might be obtained by music, diet, understanding dreams, and meditation that led to stability of the union between psyche and soma.

Plato, one of the most important figures of eastern thought in the mid-fourth century AD, recognized the primary role of medicine among the Greeks, and often alluded to the methods of the doctors in his Dialogs. If, in *Phaedo*, he stated that medicine should be an object of total man, and that a cure must direct the soul, in *Charmides* Socrates makes these ideas even more clear in his discussion with Critias:

> as you ought not to attempt to cure the eyes without the head, or the head without the body, so neither ought you to attempt to cure the body without the soul; and this, he said, is the reason why the cure of many diseases is unknown to the physicians of Hellas, because they are ignorant of the whole, which ought to be studied also; for the part can never be well unless the whole is well . . . And therefore if the head and body are to be well, you must begin by curing the soul; that is the first thing. And the cure, my dear youth, has to be effected by the use of certain charms, and these charms are fair words; and by them temperance is implanted in the soul, and where temperance is, there health is speedily imparted, not only to the head, but to the whole body . . . Let no one persuade you to cure the head, until he has first given you his soul to be cured by the charm. For this, he said, is the great error of our day in the treatment of the human body, that physicians separate the soul from the body.
>
> (Plato, 380 BCE)

The importance that Plato attributed to the noetic value of words and to the receptivity of the same by the patient is clear. In another text, his insights as to the notion of a placebo are marked. We might say that traditional psychotherapy associates to Plato through the emphasis that he gave to words in the process of a cure.

In the same period, over 200 temples of incubation dedicated to the god Aesculapius spread throughout Greece, Italy, and Turkey. Without a doubt, these were the forerunners of modern holistic treatment. A global vision of humanity predominated at these centers, and treatment was carried out by means of special baths, theater, medicinal herbs, sleep, and interpretation of dreams, all in a beautiful, pleasing environment (Solié, 1976).

Hippocrates of Cós, in the fifth century BCE, was from a family of several generations of physicians and members of the Circle of Aesculapius, and is today regarded as the father of medicine. With his observations and deductions, Hippocrates gave rise to modern medicine; words had a lower status in therapeutic methods. The rational attitude and therapy oriented by causality, with new methods for observation and treatment, took the place of the value of words.

Hippocrates regarded the brain as a receptor of phlegm, a redundant mixture liberated to relieve the body of extra heat. The heart was regarded as the seat of the soul. To Hippocrates, "anger contracted the heart, raised the heat, and carried the fluids to the head; whereas a peaceful mind, euthymia, expanded the heart" (Simms, 1980).

If we take these observations not in the concrete, physiological sense, but in a symbolic sense, we will see how correct they are. These are the expressions of feelings and of sensation from the point of view of the subject who experiences cardiac alterations. However, depreciation of the verbal mode limited the possibility of correct guidance between psyche and soma – the basis of psychosomatics.

Greek science was the start, therefore, of types of methods that were to become standard procedures in the medicine and psychology of our era. There was one great difference, however: the greater purpose was the search for knowledge of nature, and not the desire to dominate or change it.

Many centuries separate us from this position. For development, it was necessary that humans divide knowledge into compartments, separating religion, philosophy, and science. This tendency grew more pronounced through the eras until in the sixteenth century, with René Descartes, it became explicit, when he made a clear distinction between mind (spirit) and matter.

The Cartesian model

The Cartesian model emphasizes that matter is reality separated from the activity of the mind, although eventually, it would be associated to it on a divine plane. The body might be compared to a machine that would function equally well for good or evil, with or without the psyche:

> I take the body to be no other than a statue or machine made of clay, which God created.
>
> (Descartes, 1971: 120)

Although Descartes did not doubt that the origins of the spirit and of matter were in a single sphere (the divine), his methods were later interpreted as proposals to render matter and the spirit irreconcilable principles.

In a revision of the Cartesian method, Brown (1990) analyzes that the reason for our having made Descartes the villain creator of dualistic thought is the difficulty, even today, of dealing with the complexity of these phenomena. In truth, when we read his *Discourse on Method* more carefully, we will see that Descartes describes mind and body as intimately related, interdependent. In Meditation VI, "Of the Existence of Material Things and of the Real Distinction between Soul and the Body of Man", he argues that the soul is not merely "lodged" in the body "as a pilot in a vehicle", but rather that "he is very intimately connected to it ... in such a way that both make up a whole" (Descartes, 1988: 63). In *Passions of the Soul*, Descartes describes a series of states of mind as proceeding from or the consequence of alterations in the body. Both to Wilson (1980) and to Brown (1990), the true Descartes described not a rupture of mind from the body, but rather interaction that exposed the deep somatic bases of the affective and perceptive states. Far from denying mind–body interaction, Descartes supported it when he specified one place in particular where mine and body interacted – the pineal gland – although he saw the body, like a machine, as functioning without the direct intervention of the soul. Experiencing a feeling would be the outcome, and not the cause, of material, somatic action. Moreover:

> Although I may have a body to which I am closely bound, however, since on one hand I have a clear distinct idea of myself, in the measure that I am but a thinking and extensive thing, and

that, on the other, I have a distinct idea of the body, in the measure that it is but an extensive item and that it does not think, it is certain that I, that is my soul whereby I am what I am, is entire and truly distinct from my body and that it may be or exist without same.

(Descartes, 1988: 66)

Probably owing to the complexity both of his thought and of the phenomenon in itself, the majority of the contemporaries and clinical successors of Descartes understood his profound philosophy but little. Descartes was to a certain extent stigmatized as a "creator" of mind–body dualism, both in the positive sense, to promote scientific thought, and in the negative sense, more prevalent in the present day, to hinder a fuller understanding of humans.

The end of the eighteenth century lent greater emphasis to reason, while "God" had something to do with words. Rationalism, the condition of accepting the knowledge verified by means of the intellect, became the first principle.

There was also an increasing tendency to separate religion from science, mysticism and beliefs from "objective" knowledge. From the psychological point of view we might say that, in the search for consensual knowledge, the collective consciousness at this time would have achieved greater separation of the ego in relation to unconscious contents.

With the separation of religious faith from reason and science, one more stage in the collective de-integration process would have been attained.

The romantic model

If in the field of science a new model was gaining strength and power, medical practice, even in the first half of the nineteenth century, followed a romantic model where state of health was attributed to the interaction of different factors. The principal source of therapeutic knowledge was the clinical observation of patients, as we may observe in countless reports of the times.

Also referred to as romantic medicine, this model contested pure rationalism with the rediscovery of the irrationality of the psyche. Human beings were thought of as a unitary, global field rather than an aggregate of particles (Gusdorf, 1984).

Disease was defined as a non-natural imbalance caused by the interaction of biological, moral, psychological, and spiritual factors. And, as such factors were very personal, physicians rarely prescribed specific treatment for one disease. On the contrary, according to the romantic model, they emphasized the idiosyncrasies of the patients in laying out plans for treatment (Rosenkrantz, 1985). Even when suffering was located in one specific organ, it was observed that the organism reacted as a whole, in the form of resonance or compensation. All bodily disease, it was believed, might express itself in disorders at the level of consciousness, in the same way as psychological diseases would belong to an organic field. Symptoms would be linked by a relationship of correspondence and of reversibility that would be beyond mechanistic interpretation.

There is, therefore, a paradigm of a unitary, organic, and mental field, with recognition of mutuality pertaining to clinical signs: "The diseases of the soul may be written on the body from a material aspect and, reciprocally, bodily disorders may have corollaries within mental space" (Gusdorf, 1984: 259). A man who was ill was regarded in his relationship with himself, with others, and with the world, integrating art, science, and religion.

It was at this time that psychiatry became definitely incorporated into medicine and, as we shall see later, this period also saw the advent of the term "psychosomatic". Philosophers such as Schelling and Carus were to influence the development of the theory of C.G. Jung, mainly as to the concepts of the collective unconscious and the Self. For example, Schelling's concept of the archetype as primordial portrayal of the organism within a functional rational unity matches the pathology of totality in therapy concerned not with applying to each symptom an appropriate medication, but rather with interpreting symptoms as symbols of a simultaneous situation for which we should utilize a global remedy (Gusdorf, 1984). These are ideas that, with better elaboration, were to become one of the bases of analytic theory.

At this time, therefore, the treatment for a specific disease varied in accordance with the circumstances of the patient. Regimes were prescribed that included medication, diets, modified behavior, and changes in residence, and implied deep knowledge of the patient. Within this model, the doctor–patient relationship had a central role, and sensitivity to psychological factors was very important. A review of the literature of the nineteenth century shows that hundreds of articles described the psychological components of somatic disease (Warner, 1986). W. Osler, an eminent nineteenth-century English doctor, stated that:

In the medicine of the future, interdependence of mind and of body is to be more fully recognized and the form whereby one may influence the other is hardly possible to imagine at the present time.

(Lipowski, 1984: 160)

The biomedical model

Reductionism, determinism and universalism

The end of the nineteenth century, however, saw the onset of much criticism of the romantic model, above all because it was predominantly empirical and did not allow any generalization. Within this model, knowledge obtained with one patient could be applied to another only in a very limited fashion, for it depended basically on clinical observation.

Little by little, the biomedical model, based above all on experimental physiology, became more influential (Myers and Benson, 1992). Disease came to be defined as a deviation from the normal, and no longer holistically as non-natural imbalance. A focus on interaction between psychological, biological, environmental and personal factors was replaced by emphasis on biological abnormality. Clinical observation was gradually superseded by the experimental approach that came to be regarded as the main source of scientific knowledge.

Emphasis on body systems as a whole was replaced by a tendency to reduce systems to smaller parts, with each subsystem considered separately. At the same time, the focus was transferred from the individual to universal aspects of pathology. Finally, materialism took the place of a former trend that had considered moral, social and psychological (non-material) factors in dealing with the patient.

Thus, a change from the romantic model to the reductionist model was inevitable. Formulating disease as a separate entity marked by a deviation from fixed physiological norms required that the body be thought about as a set of related, though relatively independent, systems.

The search for specific etiology directed this trend even further towards reductionism, because it sought the discovery of one single specific cause of disease, rather than leading the patient to the restoration of balance. In addition, reductionism was indispensable to experimentation in a laboratory that demanded that a system be controlled by one or a few variables. This afforded conclusions on the contribution that each part made towards the whole, for here the functions of the total organism could be extrapolated and understood by an analysis of its lesser parts.

The trend towards universalism – emphasis on those aspects of disease that were universal – was also inevitable. With the acceptance of a biomedical model, the norms for countless physiological (temperature, arterial pressure, etc.) and psychological (sensations, thoughts, emotions) parameters were described. Reference to the patient as an individual was set aside because it was believed that these norms were essentially universal and, thus, deviation from them would be regarded as a disease. Measures, tests and diagnoses could be done without considering social, moral, and psychological characteristics of the patient. In this way, the practice of focusing on specific qualities of the patient was discouraged. Psychic and social factors were regarded as "epiphenomenon" with no impact on the body and, therefore, were left out of the clinical treatment.

The biomedical model also incorporated strong materialism. Nonmaterial factors were not susceptible to being easily measured in the laboratories and were thus neglected (Myers and Benson, 1992). If the "ideas" did not have "material" power, they would not be taken into account, because they would not have any effect on the body (Foss and Rothenberg, 1987).

The study of the semiology of disease, i.e. the science of the signs of a disease is from this period. The signs were no longer seen as the symbols of a disease, but rather as external manifestations of a disease. Descriptions of color, smell, sound, consistency, temperature, physical dimensions, etc. led to greater objectification reinforced by the development of technology. Here, mind and behavior were observed as quasi-physical entities, divided into sensations, ideas, feelings, for they had a place of representation in the brain and were measurable (Fabrega, 1990).

In addition, each disease began to be seen as having different patterns of development. At first, it was thought that these standards were made up of anatomical and physiological lesions. Only later, in differentiating "internal" from "external" signs, were "psychological lesions" thought of, as in neurosis or hallucinatory phenomena. The elaboration of a concept of hallucination and neurosis as phenomena that were "internal" and psychological in origin contributed to the distinction between that which is "purely" psychological and that which is "purely" physiological, and to the development of psychopathology (Fabrega, 1990). This distinction between abnormal states of body and mind would later lead to the concept of psychosomatics.

The semiologic approach to the study of diseases, both physical and mental, was also used in the phenomena referred to today as psychosomatic, such as a state of chronic fatigue. For example, exhaustion of unknown organic cause was and still is regarded by many clinicians as a sign of depression and, therefore, not as "real exhaustion". The complaint of organic disease without a biological basis is even today regarded as false by traditional medicine. It is left to one side or reduced to a phenomenon that is "purely" psychological and, consequently, of "less worth".

In conclusion, as we enter the twenty-first century with a fragmented vision of humanity, the emphasis on studying disease is on compartmentalization, objectivity, the concrete, and standardization. The determining myth is that which tells us that humans may dissect, manipulate and dominate nature. These factors have shaped our concept of disease and of the mind–body relationship, also laying a basis for the concept of psychosomatics.

The psychosomatic concept

Both in the field of medicine and in that of psychology, there is considerable misunderstanding as to the concept of the psyche–body relationship with disease. Concepts such as hysteria, conversion mechanisms, somatization, and psychosomatization have been used with the same significance in different articles. In dealing with empirical research the problem is aggravated, as we shall see. Many authors seem not to be concerned with definitions or theories, and conduct an empirical study without defining the concept employed. Even when the term "psychosomatic" is used, there is no consensus as to its meaning.

Historically, it seems that the first time this term was used was in 1808 by a German psychiatrist, Heinroth, in attempting to explain the origin of insomnia. Later, it was adopted (but rarely) by German and English doctors (Lipowski, 1984). According to Heinroth:

> As a general rule, the origin of insomnia is psychosomatic, but it is possible that each phase of life may, in itself, supply the complete reason for insomnia.
>
> (Margetts, 1950: 403)

Later, in 1828, Heinroth introduced the term "somato-psychic". While the latter was applied to diseases where the organic factor affected the emotional, "psychosomatic" indicated the power of "amorous passion over tuberculosis" (Haynal and Pasini, 1983).

It is considered today that Deutsch in 1922 was the first author to introduce the term "psychosomatic medicine", although it was Dunbar (1935) that provided the principal base for the formation of this area with systematic observations and the application of scientific methodology. Although Dunbar herself did not consider the term adequate because it did not express the fact that mind and body are aspects of a fundamental unit, in the absence of a better option gained currency in the public and scientific domains. Dunbar, who was influenced by Jung and Deutsch, founded the American Psychosomatic Society and its journal in 1939 (Editors, *Psychosomatic Medicine*, 1939).

Shortly before writing her book, Dunbar visited Deutsch in Vienna and Jung in Zurich (Kornfeld, 1990). Jung was at this time involved with studies to test psychophysiological reactions resulting from activation of the complexes, and also with the study of typology and physical manifestations. He states:

> The distinction between mind and body is an artificial dichotomy, an act of discrimination based far more on the peculiarity of intellectual cognition than on the nature of things. In fact, so intimate is the intermingling of bodily and psyche traits that not only can we draw far-reaching inferences as to the constitution of the psyche from the constitution of the body, but we can infer from psychic peculiarities the corresponding bodily characteristics.
>
> (Jung, 1971: 916)

On her return from the United States, Dunbar continued the studies that became a stimulus to founding of the Society, which is still probably one of the largest and strongest in this area. In the editorial of the first issue of *Psychosomatic Medicine* (1939) we have the following definition, which remains uncontested and has guided the work of this group:

> Its objective is to study the interrelation of the psychological and physiological aspects of normal and abnormal function of the body and integrate the somatic therapy in psychotherapy.
>
> (Editors, 1939: 3–5)

The publication of Dunbar's book, followed by the founding of this Society and of the journal, are regarded as marking the emergence of the field of psychosomatics as an organized field of scientific research, and gave rise to a movement intended to transform clinical attendance. However, as we have seen, in defining the field of psychosomatic medicine the editors of this journal positioned it as the interrelationship between psychological and physiological aspects of the functions of the "body". This is a biased affirmation and yet, at the same time, proposes the application of an organic approach in psychotherapy. In another passage in this article, the editors emphasize mind–body dualism in proposing that this field be separate from psychiatry and, we might add, from psychology, all of which exacerbated the mind–body dissociation (Lipowski, 1984). At this time, researchers from other areas developed similar studies demonstrating the mind–body relationship, according to the scientific parameters of the time.

In the 1930s, studies in psychophysiology developed by Pavlov and Cannon became an integral component of psychosomatics in focusing on the mechanisms that related the psychological variables to bodily functions. However, in applying classical experimental methodology, they also reinforced the dualistic view.

The Gestalt psychology of Kohler, Koffka, and Wertheimer in the 1920s and 1930s arose as a reaction to this experimental and laboratory psychology, with the thesis that the body could not be understood from the study of its isolated parts, but only as an irreducible totality with laws of its own (Heidbreder, 1964). According to Kohler, the function of each element would depend on the structure of the whole and on the laws that rule it (Kohler, 1947). As we shall see, this idea was taken up once more in the present-day holistic model.

Another important contribution to the area was that of Selye (1956) with his discovery of the syndrome of general adaptation, today more commonly known as stress syndrome. Selye defined stress as "the sum of all the non specific effects of the factors (normal activity, disease producers, drugs, etc.), which can act upon the body" (Selye, 1956: 42). "Stress is a condition, a state and although as such it is imponderable, that it manifests itself by measurable changes in the organs of the body" (Selye, 1956: 43). "Stress is usually the outcome of a struggle for self-preservation (the homeostasis) of parts within a whole" (Selye, 1956: 253).

Although his approach and research clearly follow a reductionist and organicist model, they lead to deeper reflection. Selye affirms that there is an element of adaptation in every disease. According to him, there is a group of diseases that he describes as diseases of adaptation, which would be defensive and adaptive reactions of the body, a blend of defense and submission. Some diseases would be caused by an excess of defense, others by an excess of bodily reactions of submission.

The basic implication of his ideas for psychosomatics is the discovery of how much and in what way the body is transformed under stress. According to Selye (1956), by "dissecting our difficulties [we may] clearly distinguish between the part acted by the stressor and . . . our adaptive measures of defense and surrender". Although he affirms that "man's ultimate aim is to express himself as fully as possible, according to his own rights" (Selye, 1956: 253), he lacked a more global theory about humanity that would allow him to bind his physiological findings to his philosophical concepts.

At the other extreme, Freud (1891/1954) studied the influence of emotion on the body with reference mainly to the role of etiology in the development of symptoms. His concepts of repression and conversion furnished the instruments that might be applied to the hypothesis of psychosomatic relationships.

To Freud (1895/1966), the hysterical symptoms appeared when the affect associated with an idea entered into conflict with the ego and was consequently repressed and discharged in somatic symptoms and innervations. Freud used the term "conversion" to refer to processes where excitement was transformed into hysterical symptoms, and "somatic compliance" to signify organic susceptibility prior or simultaneous to the trauma that would serve as a "bed" to hysterical conversion. However, he confined these hypotheses to hysteria and did not extend them to organic disease.

In presenting a formal theory of the unconscious within the scientific frame of reference of his times, Freud suggested that the psyche had a specific measurable topography and activities. Freudian thought also led to an explanation of the development and dynamics of culture. His theories of instincts, repression, guilt, and sublimation formed the basis for a theory on social life and on society. To him, instincts were primary forces in human life and the function of an individual would be to attain a balance between these forces and the external world, owing to the demands of the superego and of the principle of reality. The individual would, therefore, repress his instinctive life and his desires so that there might be integration on the social level, which, in turn, generates anxiety and mental disease.

Any emotional transaction would be a psychological dealing, not a question of liberty or moral freedom. Freud could not admit that these essential transactions would come from the spiritual man, not in a struggle against himself, but in search of significance. While Freud discovered the unconscious, he overestimated his power and limited its expression.

According to this focus, therapy allows the psyche to attain individual accommodation with one's condition of life, lending one greater energy, but without giving one the reason to employ it. In believing that the origin of religious thought was the expression of psychic dependence, linked to the need to diminish fear of the unknown, Freud intended to liberate humans from repressive fear dictated by religious institutions, believing that they could thus accept the finality of death and the absence of a spiritual force with equanimity. This was one of the points that led to the historical rupture with his disciple Jung.

Owing to the fertile development of psychoanalysis in this period, most of the scholars of psychosomatics up to the end of the 1940s based their studies on this approach. The most significant example is the development of the School of Chicago under the direction of Franz Alexander and Thomas French.

Alexander was strongly influenced by psychoanalysis, by Gestalt psychology and by advances in neurology and endocrinology. Although he considered that somatic and psychological phenomena occurred in the same organism, and were merely two aspects of the same process, he did not escape in practice from a dualistic vision:

> Psychosomatic research deals with processes in which certain links in the causal chain at the present stage of our knowledge lend themselves more promptly to study by psychological rather than physiological methods, in that a detailed investigation of the emotions as brain processes are not sufficiently advanced. Even when the physiological base of the psychological phenomena is better known, we can probably not do without the psychological study.
>
> (Alexander, 1923/1989: 47)

Alexander worked with the hypothesis of specificity of the disease according to which "the physiological responses to emotional, normal and morbid stimuli, vary in accordance with the nature of the emotional state that unleashes them" (Alexander, 1923/1989: 55). There

would be a specificity (organic) in the manner whereby a psychological motivating force might express itself (Alexander, 1923/1989:
57). Thus, each disease would correspond to an emotional picture or
to a type of personality. Alexander described seven diseases later
known as psychosomatic, but he considered that "every disease is
psychosomatic since the emotional factors influence all of the processes of the body, by means of nervous and humoral routes"
(Alexander, 1923/1989: 44).

Although the concept follows a linear, causal, and reductivistic
model, Alexander made extremely significant descriptions and clinical analyses, particularly if they are interpreted in the light of a
broader theory.

Within the psychoanalytical line, another outstanding contribution is that of the Psychosomatic School of Paris through Marty,
M'Uzan and David (1963). Here, the central idea is that psychosomatic patients differ from others by the poverty of their symbolic
world. They dream little and their dreams are "realistic". There is
little psychic elaboration and their thought is of the operatory type,
imprisoned in concrete and in pragmatic orientation. A psychosomatic patient would have little connection with his unconscious
mind. In the face of any stress on the part of the patient, through
incapacity to symbolize he would react with somatic disease. These
authors state that organic diseases, unlike neuroses and psychoses,
lack any sense and have no symbolic significance, with psychic and
organic disease being incompatible.

Sífneos and Nehemiah developed a similar idea regarding the concept of alexithymia in 1970.[1] To them psychosomatic patients would
be alexithymic, i.e. incapable of defining and expressing feelings, and
having difficulty in recognizing feelings (Sífneos and Nehemiah,
1970).

In spite of the heuristic worth of this concept, it has had limited
acceptance, as it goes against most of the clinical observations of
professionals:

> In practice, however, we see psychosomatic manifestations
> develop into hysterical, obsessive and psychotic persons. We can
> see psychosomatic symptoms being incorporated to significant
> associative chains in neurotics or articulated to deliria in psy-
> chotic persons, although we also observe the existence of patients
> classically somatizing, as per Marty.
>
> (Santos and Otelo 1992: 110)

The problem in psychoanalytical conceptualism in psychosomatics is to work with a symbol only on the verbal, abstract plane. In considering that somatization does not have a symbolic significance, and is but a signal of a dysfunction, the French School loses a direct route for work with the unconscious and gives rise to a technical difficulty. Thus, Marty (1990) proposes to psychoanalysts a therapeutic non-psychoanalytical form of work, such as using relaxation techniques for somatizing patients.

Although the psychoanalyst McDougall (1986, 1989) refers to these alexithymic patients as normopaths, i.e. those that use false non-affective normality in order to adapt, she considers that many organic patients are not within the framework of this approach and, as we shall see, she makes some valuable observations.

We shall see, therefore, that many ideas were developed without a coherent framework that would group them and that would afford coherence between theory and therapeutic practice.

According to Mello *et al.* (1992), psychosomatics has evolved in three phases:

(a) initial or psychoanalytical, with a predominance of studies on the unconscious genesis of diseases, on the theories of regression, and on secondary benefits in falling ill, among others
(b) intermediary or behaviorist, characterized by stimulus to research in men and animals, in an attempt to frame the findings in the light of exact sciences and lending great stimulus to studies on stress
(c) actual or multidisciplinary in which the importance of the social and of psychosomatic vision as an activity essentially of interaction emerges with interconnections among several health professionals (Mello *et al.*, 1992: 19).

We could add that in the third phase, where we are now, there is not a coherent theory. The model that we still use follows the classical biomedical model.

In the words of Castiel:

> The trail to be followed in search of a proposal that is more consistent for constitution of a paradigm that produces more effective psychosomatic interventions must include theoretical developments, in such a way as to reverse the ideology of a scientific medicine man that has permeated medicine and that originates in the positivist tradition of the XIX century. In this

way, medical thought is impregnated with the curative model . . .
We thus resort to interventions that have had an important degree
of effectiveness, but that now, besides producing considerable
iatrogenic effects, are not so effective.

(Castiel, 1991: 272)

We may observe, therefore, that the concept of psychosomatization,
although it represents a new de-integration in the collective consciousness, is still immersed in the biomedical model, which may be
summarized as follows: the body is a machine that must be analyzed
and reduced to its smallest parts. Psyche and body have a causalistic
and deterministic relationship and it is possible to differentiate them
objectively. Health is defined as absence of disease, which, in turn, is
defined as poor function of the biological and/or psychological
mechanisms.

Since the 1980s this model has begun to lose strength and has,
in some sectors, been replaced by the so-called holistic model. This,
as we shall see, partly encompasses the romantic model, has a
parallel in the development of contemporary science and includes a
vision of an ecological and all-inclusive world whereby the universe
is seen as a live interconnected system.

As Campbell says:

New myths have arisen from the idea that man came from the
earth and was not thrown here from somewhere . . . man is the
earth, is the conscience, the eyes and the voice of the earth . . .
All of the planet is one single organism.

(Campbell, 1990: 25)

Up to the present time, no conceptual or institutional theoretical
frame of reference has been established that may situate the problem
of health and disease within a new paradigm. We must, therefore,
gradually formulate a new theoretical approach and develop methods
of research and treatment accordingly.

The holistic model

Indeterminability, relativism and pluralism

"Holistic" is a word that comes from the Greek *holos* (whole).
According to Weil, it was first used in science in 1926 by Smuts in the

book *Holism and Evolution* to designate the concept that the universe is in constant formation. A vital force is responsible for the formation of complexes on different levels: ideological, biological, and psychological (Weil, 1990).

To Smuts, totality is a fundamental characteristic of the universe; product of a propulsion to synthesize that comes from nature. "Holism creates itself and its final structures are more holistic than its initial structures" (Ferguson, 1980: 156). Therefore, totalities are dynamic, evolutionary and creative. They cannot be understood by dissection into parts. They cannot be predicted by observation of their components. Many years passed before the term "holism" could be incorporated in different areas of knowledge.

Progress in molecular medicine, in neurobiology, in genetics, and in the application of quantum theory in biology has broadened our manner of seeing the mind–body relationship and has led to new reflections on health and on disease. Modern scientific thought, in physics and chemistry as in biology and psychology, has led us to a vision of the world that is, to a certain extent, close to that of more traditional and "natural" cultures. Thus, new trends have begun to posit a holistic principle or psychic force greater than any neurobiological event, and the molecular descriptions of psychic life have begun to reveal mind–body interdependence as a significant unit.

Quantum physics has taught us that matter and energy are two different aspects of the same reality, and that their physical characteristics may be observed only as statistical probability. This indeterminability is, in fact, a function of the matter–energy relationship with the mind of an experimenter. Therefore, quantum theory questions the principles of causality and determinism, leading to deep changes both in human and in biological sciences, just as in the theory of evolution and in psychology. Within this paradigm, vital force (like gravitational force, among others) cannot be known reductively. We can measure their effects, but in essence they are non-demonstrable.

If the molecular level is useful for the study of physiological events, it is on the quantum level that matter and psyche meet. Modern science thus suggests the problematical nature of knowledge and leaves to one side the idea of a consensual, normative, objective world.

Here, the idea of normal and universal is questioned. Martins and Bicudo state that:

Just as the position or momentum of a particle, the motivations and attitudes of an individual are not objects that present characteristics that can be objectively measured; rather, such characteristics are related to the place, moment, manner, and to why they were measured.

(Martins and Bicudo, 1989: 69)

Laszlo (1993), one of the most prominent scientists of our era, in his quest for a unified theory affirms that science is on the threshold of another "revolution" that promises to be even vaster than the Copernican revolution, and it can only unfold across the disciplines as a more holistic, systemic approach, as a cosmological revolution, in the sense in which cosmology has always been the science of the whole of reality.

In the field of psychosomatics we find some publications that attempt to integrate these concepts within a new definition:

> Psychosomatic is a term that refers to the inseparability and interdependence of the psychological and biological aspects of humanity. This connotation may be referred to as holistic, in that it implies a vision of human beings as a totality, a mind–body complex immersed in a social environment.

(Lipowski, 1984: 167)

According to Capra (1982), a holistic approach in health and in cure is in harmony with many more traditional points of view, and is also consistent with modern scientific theories.

In medicine and in psychology the term "psychosomatic" has been used, as we have seen, to refer to a disease without a diagnosis that is clearly organic. The modern use of the term has become modified. It derives from the knowledge of a fundamental interdependence between mind and body in all of the stages of sickness and health. It would be reductionism to consider that there are diseases caused only by psychological or organic factors. There are always many variables involved in the observation of any phenomenon. Thus, we should regard all diseases as psychosomatic, in so far as they involve continuous interrelation between body and mind in their origin, development, and cure.

LeShan (1992), an eminent psychologist and researcher in this area, has described the three principles that support modern psychosomatic medicine. The first states that an individual exists on many levels or domains, all of equal importance. To divide them into body, mind and spirit has been most common in the Western tradition; however, other levels may also be used. Second, each person may be seen as unique and treated as such. And third, the patient must be encouraged to benefit from his/her autonomy in the process of cure.

According to these three principles, we may help to develop an environment where the abilities of individuals to cure themselves will more probably surface to assist an allopathic medical program. From another point of view, we may say that these principles tend to produce a superior level of activity in the processes and structures that we refer to as "the immunological system", for example. Here it is important to remember that any system is an offshoot (i.e. "de-integrated") that is somewhat arbitrary, and that does not have, as such, an absolute truth. With other offshoots, other laws have been discovered; systems that are very different from those with which we are accustomed would probably have been developed in different circumstances. The medicine–psychology division is one of these "de-integrated" systems that will certainly be outdated at some time in the future.

In conclusion, a new synthesis is necessary. A new de-integration begins to emerge from the collective unconscious, forming a new model. Our evolution depends on the level of our consciousness and on our capacity to bring forth the information that is already in the unconscious.

The holistic model, in resuming former concepts, practices, methods, and techniques, tries to integrate them in the modern world. However, we can observe, even among the authors that use a new approach, the absence of a conceptual model. The diverse researchers and clinicians in the area, including LeShan, have not defined the theoretical paradigm that underpins them. Techniques are applied and tested, in general with good results, but in a form that is eminently empirical.

On the other hand, on brief reflection, we can see that this new attitude and the new approach are described completely in analytical psychology. The principles of the holistic model, as described above, are found in the theory and in the psychotherapy method proposed by Jung, even if the latter has not contributed directly to the former.

Therefore, our proposal is to use the analytic model to develop a theory applicable to the phenomenon of disease and health, in its interrelation with the psyche–body phenomenon.

Chapter 2

The analytical model

Our brains deal exclusively with special-case experiences. Only our minds are able to discover the generalized principles operating without exception in each and every special-experience case which if detected and mastered will give knowledgeable advantage in all instances.

(Fuller, 1963: 1)

The psychophysical experiments

Although references to the body/mind issue are rare in analytical psychology, by 1906 Jung had already laid the foundation for considering this phenomenon by developing the word association test.

Initially used to diagnose neuroses and psychoses through the complexes that surfaced during the experiment, and to shorten the time of "psychoanalysis", this experiment proved to be an area for basic observation of human psychophysiology. Jung was speaking of the these tests' results when he said:

Physical and psychic symptoms are nothing more than symbolic manifestations of pathogenic complexes.

(Jung, 1973: 727)

Through these experiments of association, Jung observed that a complex works as an automaton and replaces the constellatory power of the egoic complex.

In this way, a new morbid personality is gradually created, the inclinations, judgments, and resolutions of which move only in the direction of the will to be ill. This second personality devours what is left of the normal ego and forces it into the role of a secondary (oppressed) complex.

(Jung, 1973: 861)

The ego [is] defined herein as nothing but a complex of imaginings held together and fixed by the coenesthetic impressions.

(Jung, 1973: 1352)

There is a similarity between the ego and the secondary complexes, for the emotional tone of these is also based on coenesthetic impressions, in the knowledge that either one or the other may be temporarily repressed or split up.

(Jung, 1973: 1352)

Countless cases and studies reported by Jung clearly established the function of a neurotic symptom as the best expression of conflict lived and repressed, mainly in hysterical patients.

In the depths of the mind of each hysterical patient we always find an old wound that still hurts or, in psychological terms, a feeling-toned complex.

(Jung, 1973: 915)

The same concept was used in the explanation of psychoses (Jung, 1973: 1353). In the Psychiatric Clinic laboratory, Jung together with Peterson carried out a wide-ranging study on psycho-physical reactions in normal and in psychopathological individuals. The purpose of these studies was:

to ascertain the value of the so-called psycho-physical galvanic reflex as a recorder of psychical stimuli; to determine its normal and pathological variations; to study the respiratory innervation curve in the same relations; and finally to compare the galvanometer and pneumograph, under the influence of various stimuli.

(Jung, 1973: 1036)

In a brief summary of Jung's discoveries, we might cite the following:

1   The fluctuation on a galvanometer and in the time of reaction may be used as a measure of amount of emotional tone. Each stimulus that accompanies an emotion precipitates an elevation

in the electrical curve that is directly proportionate to the vivacity and actuality of the emotion elicited (Jung, 1973: 1049).

2   An emotion imagined may produce the same reactions (Jung, 1973: 1050).

3   Great emotional liability precipitates a considerable variation in the curves of a pneumograph and galvanometer (Jung, 1973: 1057).

4   Breathing is subject to a process of inhibition in the presence of expectation, tension, and emotion; however, because it is more subject to conscious control, sometimes the pneumographic curve does not show a marked change (Jung, 1973: 1062).

5   Alterations in breathing owing to emotional states are more marked in breathing out, at the moment of relaxation, than during breathing in (Jung, 1973: 1063).

6   The time elapsed between one stimulus and the change in electrical resistance of the skin, as shown by the galvanometer, suggest alterations in the sympathetic nervous system, probably under the influence of the sudoriferous glands (Jung, 1973: 1064).

7   The galvanometer curve for these reasons is more intimately connected than the pneumographic curve with the emotional complexes (Jung, 1973: 1064).

The association experiments furnished a means for experimental study of the behavior of complexes and of the psyche–body relation, enabling better comprehension of the ego's structure and the personal unconscious.

The theory of complexes

Thus, a complex was conceived by Jung as:

> a collection of imaginings, which, in consequence of this autonomy, is relatively independent of the central control of the consciousness, and at any moment liable to bend or cross the intentions of the individual.
>
> (Jung, 1973: 1352)

For Jung, both in neuroses and in psychoses, symptoms of a somatic or psychic nature originate in the complexes. In neuroses, the complexes undergo continual changes, while in the psychoses they remain fixed, preventing the personality from progressing (Jung, 1973: 1354). The more intense and more autonomous the complex, the greater the symptomology: "a strong complex possesses all the characteristics of a separate personality" (Jung, 1973: 1352).

Through innumerable research studies, Jung demonstrated that the basis both of the ego and of the secondary complex is the body, insofar as both have their emotional tone based on coenesthetic impressions, understood here as the totality of sensations that originate in the body organs, i.e. sensations through which the body itself is perceived.

Elaborating later (1974), Jung makes it clear that the ego, originating in the Self archetype, has one psychic basis and another somatic. The somatic basis would consist of the conscious and unconscious endosomatic sensations. The emergence of the ego would be touched off by the "collision between the somatic factor and the environment" (Jung, 1974: 3–6).

Fordham (1957), through clinical research on children, also demonstrated that the ego originates from the totality archetype, the Self, which expresses itself, as do all archetypes, in body experience on the one hand, and in archetypal images on the other.

Thus when a given complex constellates, there is not only a change on the physiological level, as shown by the association experiments, but also a transformation in the total body structure, whether or not the individual realizes it. This transformation may be felt as an indefinite sense of ill-being or may express itself in clearer symptoms.

So we may note that every complex, including the ego complex, has a specific pattern of coenesthetic images and sensations. The body self-image is part of the ego complex, just as are all coenesthetic sensations consciously present, forming a consistent and relatively stable structure in the normal individual.

The formation of the symbol

The formation of the body image is not merely the result of personal experiences, but is based on the ego–Self relation, which has its own bodily representation. Body consciousness is "de-integrated"; it is the perception of a part of the total body, of the corporeal Self.

The development of individual and/or collective consciousness brings to the surface other new "de-integrateds", other knowledge, that is joined to this forever partial perception of the body consciousness. Knowledge of the total body would correspond to knowledge of Self's body, of Totality's body.

To the normal individual the de-integrated arises in consciousness as a symbol, sometimes in its more concrete pole, other times in its more abstract pole, but always acting synchronistically in the two cases. The development of the ego depends in part on its ability to absorb these symbols, images, and sensations that supply the ego with information about the Self.

For their part, the Self's symbols emerge from the depths of the body. Jung says:

> The symbol is thus a living body, *corpus et anima* . . . The deeper layers of the psyche lose their individual uniqueness as they retreat farther and farther into darkness . . . Lower down, that is to say as they approach the autonomous functional systems, they [the symbols] become increasingly collective until they are universalized and extinguished in the body's materiality, i.e., in chemical substances. The body's carbon is simply carbon. Hence "at bottom" the psyche is simply "world" . . . The more archaic and deeper, that is the more *physiological*, the symbol is, the more collective and universal, the more "material" it is.
>
> (Jung, 1974: 29)

Starting from these statements, we might inquire whether the more a disease manifests itself in the body, the more it is an expression of the collective and universal unconsciousness. Here the question would be: is a disease that has a clearly corporeal representation expressing content more unconscious, more collective? Can it be that those patients considered more "psychosomatic" are expressing contents more archaic than those patients who are less sick physically?

When we compare these patients with psychotics, we see that the latter also express decidedly archaic and archetypal contents and that therefore the difference must not be one of the degree of primitivism and lack of differentiation, but perhaps one of the quality of the psychotics' expression. While psychotic manifestation occurs mainly on the abstract level, the "organic" invalid expresses himself mainly on the concrete level. Perhaps the difference lies in the way of expressing this structuring, since both may be manifesting disorganization or non-differentiation of a primary level. Thus, we may reason that while in psychosis the ego is menaced with extinction by invading archetypal contents, in cancer (for example) the organism, including the ego, is being threatened with extinction by "invading cells that proliferate indiscriminately."

Another way to formulate the question would be: is the conflict that finds expression in abstract symbols (fantasies, dreams, imagination) closer to consciousness than that which finds more pronounced expression in the organic aspect? If it is, the idea of alexithymia makes some sense. In the absence of an abstract symbolic representation, the Self would manifest by creating more regressive, primitive, and organismic symbols. This idea has support in the thesis developed by J. Conger, who (with reference to Jung) states that:

> Symbols either reflect the archaic physiology of the body or are more differentiated, reflecting the more conscious character.
>
> (Conger, 1988: 185)

In clinical practice, however, many "organically" ill patients do not demonstrate themselves to be alexithymics nor to be reduced to operational thinking.

We cannot here reduce symbol to the verbal, as does the Psychosomatic School of Paris. That a patient somatizes, as we shall see, does not mean he does not symbolize, but rather that this symbolizing happens on the somatic plane. It would be highly reductionist to restrict the symbolization process to the verbal or abstract level.

The problem probably lies in the interconnection of conscious and unconscious life. The patient who expresses himself somatically has lost his body's connection with his somatic unconsciousness, so that his eidetic fantasy life would be disconnected from his organic life. That is to say, these patients have a more restricted and compulsive symbolic life.

Perhaps we are dealing here with archaic forms of psychic functioning: pre-verbal symbolic forms, natural at the infantile stage. Although a technical review of personality development is beyond the scope of this work, some observations are needed.

The development of the symbolic process

We know that babies react bodily to fear of, or the sensation of, being abandoned. The psychic structures are at first constructed of psychophysiological reactions. We can suppose that when an adult reacts with a physical symptom to feeling abandoned, he is re-experiencing an infantile pattern of behavior, as a child responds psychosomatically to emotional pain for lack of verbal language.

Jacoby (1999), in his study of the development of the symbolic function, describes the infant experiences as:

> a whole spectrum of body sensations; and with them, different patternings of psychophysiologycal rhythm, having to do not only with its own and its mother's heartbeat, but also with the cycle of biological and emotional states that the newborn goes through during a twenty-four hour period.
>
> (Jacoby, 1999: 62)[1]

When the mother–child relationship is sufficiently good, there will develop in the child, starting from the initial somatopsychic matrix, a progressive discrimination between his body and the mother's body, which is the first representation of the external world. The psychological contents are slowly discriminated from the somatic in the infant psyche. In the normal pattern, it is through the relation with the mother that verbal symbolic communication develops in harmony with, and complementing, corporal communication. Psyche–body differentiation grows more solid, and the mother–child relationship offers the basis for forming the transcendent function. The archetypes proceed to de-integrate as their two poles become conscious.

Also according to Jacoby, thinking and fantasizing are possible only after the emergence of the capacity of symbolizing, which occurs after the age of 18 months. And the development of this capacity "depends largely on a facilitating mirroring and an optimal dose of stimulation coming from the environment" (Jacoby, 1999: 71).

> Infants may experience states of bliss or anguish but they have no image or concept of those states. This actually makes the emotional experience, raw and unmediated as it is, much more intense and pervasive, and therefore in greater need of being contained by the caretaker.
>
> (Jacoby, 1999: 59)

In adult life, we may suppose that the difficulty in symbolizing at the most abstract level would be a consequence of prematurely interrupting the relationship to the caregiver, regardless of the reason. Thus fear, rather than transforming into a mental process, would get stuck on the physical plane.

Although the organic patient may function rather well in certain personality areas, in some patients it is possible to see a split between body and psyche. How exactly this happens, we do not yet know. Nevertheless, we know that it is the mother, or a substitute, who decodes for the child, verbally and with gestures, both external stimuli and his apparent corporal sensations. In this context the mother would thus function as a protector and decodifier, carrying out the transcendent function for the child. It is through this relationship that the child learns to identify his body abstractly.

If certain emotional states cannot be elaborated with abstract symbols, they may became isolated fragments of a purely concretized nature (Jacoby, 1999: 66) and a split would tend to occur. This split, according to McDougall, might be resolved in two ways:

> The first leads to autistic pathology, in which case the body and its somatic functioning frequently remain intact while the mind closes itself to the external world; the second keeps the relation to external reality intact, with the risk that the soma will begin to act in what we might call an "autistic" fashion, that is, detached from the psyche's affective messages in terms of word-presentations, leaving powerful thing-presentations to seek non-verbal expression.
>
> (McDougall, 1989: 43)

Thus we might reason that in these patients a complex has no way to be represented on an abstract level and therefore cannot be expressed through fantasy, imagination, or dreaming. But this conflict may indeed take on an organic expression. In this way, the organic symptom will contain psychic messages that otherwise would have no abstract representation.

McDougall observes that organic patients "resist the search for the psychic factors that nourish their psychosomatic vulnerability" (McDougall, 1989: 43). It is as if these patients struggle, as do neurotic and psychotic patients, to protect their somatic creation.

Fordham (1957) developed a similar idea. According to this author, the mother, by not mediating for the child between psyche and body, keeps the symbolic, transcendent function locked in the body, rather than its changing into fantasies and images that would be assimilated by the ego. It's as if the emotional memory got lost in the body and reappeared when current situations mirrored a conflict similar to that which gave rise to this split. The archetype's two poles are split. There is no space to symbolize emotional pain verbally; that's why it is experienced in the body. In this case, somatization would be acting out and trying to integrate the repressed instinct (archetype) into consciousness. But due to difficulty in expressing at a more conscious level, the corporal symptom keeps repeating compulsively and defensively.

This hypothesis has been confirmed by innumerable clinical cases, where the sentiment of fear does not accompany the normally concomitant physiological sensation. That is, the patient complains of organic symptoms without being aware that they refer to a certain conflictive sentiment. For example, a patient who had tachycardiac and hypertensive crises took some time to see that they were concomitant to the sentiment of panic (appearance of a complex).

The issue of why a person with a conflict reacts neurotically, whereas another reacts with a somatic disease, is far from being answered. Some hypotheses, however, have been broached. Here it is also necessary to discriminate between the causes that precipitate the symptom and the psychic organizational structure that reacts somatically in face of a conflict. Hundreds of studies on stress fall into the first of these categories.

In summary, one of the hypotheses we could raise would be that psychosomatic phenomena may be avoided when neurotic forms of organization emerge. The neurotic structure creates a protective structure, namely the neurotic symptom, to deal with the conflict or emotional pain, whereas in organic disturbances there would be a regression to more primitive forms of relationship between body and mind. The verbal communication of affective states would be disconnected, in general, from the body. Here an archaic form of symbolism is at work, in which the body talks. A symptom that may be corporal ("organic illness") or psychic ("mental illness") would be the symbolic representation of a disconnection or disturbance in the ego/Self axis.

In this context, we have to be careful about the observation, common among psychologists and doctors, that diseases of the immunological system, especially cancer, occur less frequently in psychotic patients, as if mental illness were an alternative to organic.

Several studies have been undertaken in an attempt to clarify this issue, with highly controversial results. For example, while some authors defend the idea that cancer (particularly lung cancer) occurs less often in patients with schizophrenia (Craig and Lin, 1981; Rice, 1979), others have observed incidence levels greater than (Ananth and Burnstein, 1977) or equal to the general population (Hussar, 1966; Odegard, 1967).

After an extensive review of the literature, Harris (1988) attributed this controversy to numerous methodological questions, including the use of antipsychotic medication, which has obviated clear results.

Mortensen (1989, 1994), one of the most prominent researchers in the field, developed a number of studies that looked at the occurrence of depression (in conjunction with some other type of problem) in schizophrenia. Most of the findings indicated a reduction in the risk of cancer in schizophrenic patients. His conclusions were based extensively on a cohort study of the Danish population, and an independent analysis of schizophrenic patients who had been admitted for the first time.

A study conducted by Gulbinat et al. (1992) found that three cities – Aarhus (Denmark), Nagasaki (Japan) and Honolulu (USA) – produced very interesting results. In Aarhus, there was a low incidence of two cancer types in particular: pulmonary and prostate. Among schizophrenic women, the risk for all types of cancer was equal to or slightly less than the risk to the general population. The results for Nagasaki and Honolulu revealed no significant difference, while the authors found a significant reduction of lung cancer in schizophrenic Danish men and women. This is important, as schizophrenics tend to be heavier smokers, smoking longer and preferring cigarettes that are heavier in tar.

The most recent study on the subject is the first study done on the US mainland. Cohen et al. (2002) demonstrated a reduced likelihood of a cancer diagnosis in persons diagnosed with schizophrenia, despite their higher rates of smoking. While the authors hypothesized that this finding is due solely to the use of neuroleptic medication, these results are similar to those observed at the turn of the twentieth century, well before this type of medication came into use.

It appears that this negative relation between schizophrenia and cancer is also found in relation to schizophrenia and rheumatoid arthritis. In an extensive review of the literature on the incidence of rheumatoid arthritis in schizophrenic patients, Eaton et al. (1992) found that although the evidence for the negative relationship of schizophrenia to rheumatoid arthritis is not conclusive, it is very strong: they found a consistently lower than expected co-occurrence of the two conditions.

In conclusion, the hypothesis that there is a negative relation between mental and organic illness remains open to question.

While the bulk of research points to a negative relation between schizophrenia and illnesses such as cancer and rheumatoid arthritis, methodological difficulties have prevented a clear conclusion on the phenomenon. As far as current wisdom goes, there is a tendency to express a dysfunction in either the psychic or the organic realm.

Some observations of an alternation between schizophrenic symptoms and cancer are found in cases described in the literature and in clinical practice. Recently, from the medical report of a schizophrenic woman, I could see the improvement of the mental symptoms, according to her psychiatrist, at the same time as a malign tumor was found. According to her nurse, the patient – a 58-year-old woman with chronic schizophrenia – was perfectly lucid during the treatment. It was only after discharge by her gynecologist that she experienced a severe recurrence of the mental disease.

Symbol as the third factor in the psyche–body phenomenon

Jung returns to the psyche–body phenomenon as symbol in his work on psychology and alchemy, in which he states that the result of alchemical endeavor should be sought neither in the body nor in the psyche, but rather

> in an intermediate realm between mind and matter, i.e. a psychic realm of subtle bodies whose characteristic it is to manifest themselves in a mental as well as a material form . . . Obviously, the existence of this intermediate realm comes to a sudden stop the moment we try to investigate matter in and for itself, apart from all projection; and it remains non-existent so long as we believe we know anything conclusive about matter or the psyche. But the moment when physics touches on the "untrodden, untreadable regions", and when psychology has at the same time to admit that there are other forms of psychic life besides the acquisitions of personal consciousness – in other words, when psychology too touches on an impenetrable darkness – then the intermediate realm of subtle bodies comes to life again, and the physical and the psychic are once more blended in an indissoluble unity.
>
> (Jung, 1968: 394)

In his work, the terms "subtle body", "pneumatic body", "breath-body" (Jung, 1970: 513; 1972: 390), "internal body" and *corpus glorificatus* are used as relatively synonymous. *Corpus subtile* is a transfigured and resurrected body, i.e. a body that was at the same time spirit (Jung, 1968: 511). *Corpus glorificatus* or *glorificationis* is the body of the resurrection, the subtle body, in the state of incorruptibility (Jung, 1975: 202), "a state achieved by the hero as reward for his victory" (Jung, 1970: 513). "It is a pure and eternal substance capable and worthy of being united with the *unio mentalis*" (Jung, 1974: 774).

The subtle body is also mixed up with the somatic unconscious. In his seminars on Nietzsche, Jung states that the unconscious can only be experienced in the body and that the body is exclusively the external manifestation of the Self (Jung, 1988).

Meir (1986), revisiting the theory of the subtle body, considers that it is in that theory that we will eventually find the solution for problems of the psychophysical relationship. The subtle body, to him, is a third factor, greater than the body and greater than the psyche, and responsible for forming symptoms in both.

Mindell (1982, 1985) develops from these concepts a new term: "dreambody". This author considers that the relation between subtle body and real body is given by the oniric body, for both the subtle and the real are aspects of the oniric body.

A similar concept is developed by Sandner (1986), who describes the subjective body as the archetype through which the psyche influences the objective (real) body, and vice versa.

This body of which these authors speak is the expression of the archetype of the original human, of his corporal schema, as Neumann (1973) says; and it is his symbolic body, according to Byington. As Byington understands it, the body participates in the psyche via the structuring symbols that express the individual's personal traits. The symbolic body is defined here as the set of psychological significance of the somatic body. Beyond this:

> every one of the five corporal systems (respiratory, digestive, cardiovascular, neuroendocrine, and motor) affects, in characteristic manner, countless symbols which typically structure our identity and our style of being and of knowing the world.
>
> (Byington, 1988: 29)

With all these conceptions, symbol comes forward as the third factor in mind–body polarity. Subtle body, pneumatic body, somatic unconscious, dreambody or oniric body, subjective body, and symbolic body are all concepts which refer to a third factor that transcends the psyche–body dichotomy: the symbol.

In summary, symbol expresses the perception of the psyche–body phenomenon by perceiving, synchronistically, physiological changes and the corresponding images. A complex always has a corporeal symbolic expression through which we may grasp the key to comprehending the illness. In the case of a complex, the symbol points toward a dysfunction, a detour that needs correction because the relation of ego to Self has changed.

In Groddeck, regarded by many as the father of psychosomatic medicine, we find the same idea. To him, disease does not exist as an entity, but only as the expression of totality of man, as an expression of "this" (id). To cure would be "to correctly interpret that which this totality is trying to express through symptoms and to teach it a less painful mode of self expression" (Groddeck, 1992: 173).

Several authors, including Reich (1954/1955), tried to establish a correlation between the organic and the psychic symptomatology based on a similar idea. However, in so far as they tried to establish fixed and universal relationships between body and mind, they brought about a rigid and reductionistic system. As we shall see, the same can be said of Temoshok and Dreher (1992) (cancer and type C personality) and Friedman and Rosenman (1974) (cardiac disease and type A personality), among others, in trying to establish a relationship between the personality traits and disease.

The transcendent function and the theory of transduction

Rossi (1986) proposes a psychobiological theory of mind/body communication, in which symbol is present through word or placebo using techniques of hypnosis. He defines the conscious as "a process of self-reflective information transduction" (Rossi, 1986: 11).

Transduction theory refers to the conversion or transformation of energy or information from one form to another. Here the human body is seen as a network of information systems (genetic, immunological, hormonal, *inter alia*). Each of these systems has its code, and the transmission of information between the systems requires some type of transducer to allow the code of one system to be translated to that of another.

The mind, with its capacity to symbolize linguistically, may also be considered as a mean of coding, processing, and transmitting the organism's, psyche's and soma's information. The organic patient would code his conflict in the somatic system, by preference.

The question then is that of how the information received and processed on the semantic level, for example, may be transduced into information appropriate to be received on the somatic level, and vice versa.

Rossi addresses this question by investigating the technique of hypnosis as facilitating the process of transducing mind/body information, based principally on studies of the limbic/hypothalamic system, which he considers the major psyche–body transducer.

The concept of symbol as "energy-transforming machine," proposed by Jung (1970), would here be comprehended as the transducing machine through which a system's information (e.g. the immunological system's) could be transduced to the conscious system, and vice versa. Rossi goes so far as to suggest that

> The successful lucid dreamer is the individual who can use a certain degree of conscious planning and voluntary control to transduce mind into physiological responses.
>
> (Rossi, 1986: 29)

That is, an individual who, besides controlling some of his oniric states, can have access to certain psychophysiological functions.

> Mind and body are presumably a pair of opposites and, as such, the expression of a single entity whose essential nature is not knowable either from its outward, material manifestation or from inner, direct perception . . . This living being appears outwardly as the material body, but inwardly as a series of images of the vital activities taking place within it.
>
> (Jung, 1972: 619)

In this sense, the symbol would be informing of organic events. This idea finds substrata in the case histories of patients who describe dreams indicative of organic diseases well before any such illnesses are perceived.

A patient of mine once dreamt that she had a clump of arteries and veins wrapped around her left foot. She woke up screaming when, in her dream, a doctor had threatened to cut the clump open.

Her associations in no way explained the meaning of this dream. Intrigued, we let it be until almost 20 days afterwards she was diagnosed with an angio-sarcoma tumor, a rare type of vein and artery cancer. It was at this time that the patient remembered the dream that had remained concealed. Another patient who dreamt of crabs crawling on her chest was immediately taken to her oncologist, where she was diagnosed with breast cancer. In this second case, the image was more easily interpreted due to the association between the words "cancer" and "crab" in the Latin language. Accordingly, more profound observations of the oniric world can allow a preliminary diagnosis – even before the visible manifestation of an illness.

The use of the transcendent function in the therapeutic process coincides with the method of transducing described above:

> to gain possession of the energy that is in wrong place, he [the patient] must make the emotional state the basis or starting point of the procedure . . . The whole procedure is a kind of enrichment and clarification of the affect, whereby the affect and its contents are brought nearer to consciousness . . . This is the beginning of the transcendent function, i.e., of the collaboration of conscious and unconscious data.
>
> (Jung, 1972: 167)

Jung continues describing various methods, denominated "amplification", by which we may make the transition (transduction) from unconscious contents, as organic or emotional symptoms, to the conscious plane – methods such as active imagination or the use of painting and clay.

Here we should remember the limits of the psychoanalytical technique in this field. In regarding the organic symptoms as pre-symbolic representations, McDougall emphasizes the therapeutic need to convey them to the verbal plane, underestimating the value of the image and thus losing valuable material (McDougall, 1989).

Synchronicity

Implicit in the concept described here of disease and symbol, we have the concept of synchronicity.

Synchronicity refers to the existence of two or more phenomena occurring at the same time, without any relationship of cause and effect between them, but with a relationship of significance. This type of phenomenon shows that the non-psychic may behave as the psychic, and that the psychic may behave as does the somatic, without there being any causal relationship between either pair.

Using this concept, we may realize more easily that an image does not cause a certain sensation and that a certain sensation does not lead to the formation of an image, but that both are simultaneously present in the organism, consciously or not. In so far as psyche and body form a pair of opposites, their relation cannot be perceived as that of cause and effect. The third – transcendent – factor that we call symbol, when it is in the conscious, reveals that "psyche and matter are two different aspects of one and the same thing" (Jung, 1972: 418).

Therefore, each and every disease finds expression in the body and the psyche simultaneously. What drives a patient to seek a doctor or a psychologist is the degree of suffering at one pole.

The finalist approach and the compensation mechanism

Jung proposes a finalist approach together with the method of amplification so that we may better understand the unconscious phenomenon. For him, the basic purpose both of neurosis and of any manifestation of the unconscious would be to compensate a unilateral attitude of consciousness, showing the attitude necessary so that the ego may integrate the repressed material.

Extending the concept of compensation to the area of organic illness, we would say that such illness is a symbolic expression that aims to compensate a one-sided attitude of the conscious. Organic illness would be the organism's reaction in compensation, with the object of forcing the individual to integrate the repressed, reconnecting the ego to its axis with the Self.

To Ziegler (1983), who developed this thesis extensively, understanding of a disease will be complete only when we leave the solid ground of empirical medicine, for:

> as experience has shown, categorizing pathologies according to disease entities does not allow for an appreciation of the mutual dynamic of health and disease.
>
> (Ziegler, 1983: 24)

We will be talking about *disease images*, not empirical constructs in which symptoms are more or less arbitrarily lumped together on basis of statistical frequency.

(Ziegler, 1983: 23)

To Ziegler, somatization would be the limit imposed by nature faced with an excess of energy channeled unilaterally. Nature counter-balances this tendency via the body, as if it sought a more effective means to realize its goals. "The insensitivity of our healths deter-mines our illnesses. Our lack of concern and attention can only go so far before meeting set limits" (Ziegler, 1983: 13).

Here, the causal factors – genetic or social, for example – are considered instruments through which the compensatory mechanism acts. An allergic reaction, for example, on handling a substance at work, may reveal an unconscious inflammatory hypersensibility to this work, expressed by the allergy. This "somatization" may then be comprehended as a form of compensation that leads the sick person to correct his exaggeratedly one-sided relationship with his environment.

Given this analytical conception, we now take up the psyche–body question again and situate it within the modern scientific holistic model.

In what follows, we will present a summary of this model, developed within analytic theory, in order to apply the model to the understanding and treatment of organic disease.

Chapter 3

Disease as symbolic expression

A new proposal

> One thing, however, I should like to ask of you, namely, to abandon the distinction between "mental" and "organic" in corresponding with me . . . in essence both mean the same, both are subject to the same laws of life, both take their root in the same life.
>
> (Groddeck, 1949: 119)

By recognizing the transcendent element, the transducer, in the psychic apparatus, analytic psychology considers once more the question of the meaning of disease, both physical and mental, and introduces a new methodology in accordance with current scientific parameters.

The concept of symbol as third factor in the psyche–body phenomenon, as well as the goal-oriented view and the compensation mechanism, complements the question of duality and of psychophysical causality and renders obsolete the term "psychosomatization". Although the use of this term may still be nearly unavoidable in clinical practice, we need to remember that its use takes us back to a classical, mechanistic, reductionist biomedical tradition. Constant effort is needed for us not to fall into a model outdated much more in theory than in practice.

For didactic purposes, we may summarize the ideas developed so far as follows.

1   The first association tests proved that every psychic phenomenon has a physiological correlate. Technical developments in physiological instrumentation have proved this fact over and over again, as have hundreds of research studies that show the relationship between stress and physiological changes.

2   Somatic or psychic symptoms may have their origin in the complexes. The constellation of a complex synchronistically triggers an alteration on the physiological and psychological levels, whether or not the individual perceives these alterations.

3   Each complex has a specific pattern of images and sensations rooted in the archetype. For this reason, the physiopathological and psychopathological manifestations of a complex exhibit a degree of universality. Compatible studies that try to correlate personality traits with disease have had interesting results: for example, personality Type A with cardiac diseases; personality Type C with diseases of the immunological system.

4   The egoic complex is formed along the length of the ego–Self axis and develops by means of a process of de-integration and of symbolic function also known as a transcendent function or transducer function. A secondary complex is a deviation in the development of the ego–Self axis and also manifests itself symbolically.

5   The archetype may be experienced as a physiological dynamism and may enter consciousness as an image, showing that psyche and body are different aspects of the archetype, because the archetype is located outside of the psychic sphere. There would be a graduation, a spectrum, with the instinctive contents at one end and the conscience at the other. The dynamism of instinct would be, as stated by Jung, in the infrared part of the spectrum, whereas the image of instinct would be in the blue part (Jung, 1972: 414). The awareness and assimilation of the instinct would never occur at the red point, i.e. by absorption on the instinctive sphere, but only through integration of the image that means and, at the same time, invokes instinct.

6   The real nature of the archetype may be transcendent: it is not to be made aware. It would be in the ultraviolet part of the spectrum, a mixture of blue and red. All we know about archetypes is behaviors, visualizations, thoughts, inferences, images or concretization that belong to the field of consciousness.

7   Both the behavioral expression of health and that of disease may be seen as symbolic representations of the relationship ego/Self.

8   Each and every symptom is a symbolic expression, a symbol that reveals a dysfunction along the ego/Self axis. An understanding of the meaning of this symbol reveals the correction to be made (compensation mechanism). In this way, we once again take up earlier models of cure without getting attached to them.

9   The symptom/symbol compensates for the "error" and synchronistically points to the "correction" to be made, i.e. what
unconscious content needs to be integrated into consciousness.

10   In the organically ill individual, coenesthetic impressions, the
bases of ego and complexes, are split from their abstract
representations.

11   We may hypothesize that the patient who expresses this dysfunction by an organic symbol has split off his fantasy life from the
coenesthetic impression, expressing himself by means of pre-
verbal symbolic functioning. Another hypothesis is that the conscious has difficulty integrating the emerging symbol due to its
complexity. We can observe that a profound or traumatic exis-
tential situation may bring about questioning that the ego is
induced to somatize when it cannot integrate the questioning on
the abstract plane.

12   The disease/symbol may be transduced into different systems, all
probably synchronistic and expressing the same archetype. To
understand the meaning of this symbol, it is not enough for us
to search for the cause; we must research into the disease's/
symbol's goal. Why? and To what end? complement one another,
enhancing our knowledge.

Note that the word "symbol" comes from the Greek *syn* (together)
+ *ballein* (to throw), which means a joining of opposites, combining
the known with the unknown, unconsciously. "Symptom" comes
from *syn* (together) + *piptō* (to fall), or "two things falling together"
(Funk and Wagnalls, 1950), while "to be a clinician" means "to bend
over the one who has fallen" (i.e. the ill, and their symptoms). To the
extent that symbol implies the union of something conscious with
something unconscious, it always stimulates "emotion" (*e + movere*),
meaning "to move" or "movement outside" of the vegetative nervous system, whether in the sympathetic or parasympathetic nervous
system. This gives us the key of psychosomatics: by using a symbol
we can reach the deep, inaccessible organic layers of the conscience.[1]

In concluding these considerations of the analytic model, we
summarize that the organic symptom may correspond to a split in
the representation of a complex/archetype, in which the abstract/
psychic part was repressed. On being disconnected from the ego, this
symptom recurs compulsively, trying to integrate into the conscious
so that the individuation process may continue.

The question that we pose here is: can it be that becoming conscious of the complex's abstract pole – in other words, transducing the symbol from its pathological organic to its psychic/abstract pole – would diminish its pathological organic expression? That is, would transduction of the symbol from its organic pole to its psychic/abstract pole bring about a waning of the organic symbol, improving the patient's health?

We know that in the treatment of neuroses and psychoses the method of amplifying on the symptom/symbol leads to an increase in the conscious and to greater integration of unconscious content into the ego, transforming the ego/Self relationship. This amplification may take place on the personal level through externalizing the symptom and through active imagination; on the collective level, this occurs through the comparative study of myths, tales, folklore, art and religion.

The proposal here, therefore, is to observe during the psychotherapeutic process the effect on the organic symptom's development of applying the analytic model. Our hypothesis is that:

1   organic disease may have a goal and a meaning
2   in some cases, this meaning is a symbol
3   understanding and integrating this symbol into the conscious leads to improvement in the general state of the patient's health.

For these observations, we shall utilize the study of research in psychosomatics, as it furnishes a basis for the observation of the psyche–body phenomenon. We shall utilize these data in the elucidation of the clinical cases presented.

Chapter 4

Critical analysis of psychosomatic research

> Nor will the quiet life be more temperate than the unquiet, seeing
> that temperance is admitted by us to be a good and noble thing,
> and the quick have been shown to be as good as the quiet.
>
> (Plato, *Charmides*: 380 BCE)

The study of the psyche–body phenomenon and how emotional experiences, personality, and lifestyle can influence health goes back, as we have seen, to ancient times. The relation of these factors with susceptibility to disease and its growth is a fact found in the most diverse clinical observations.

As noted above, however, the discovery approximately a century ago of pathogenic agents as a cause of infectious diseases led the principal focus of research to the biomedical and pharmacological model. Only in the past 30 years has there been a progressive and accelerated resurgence of interest in the emotional factors in diseases in general – primarily among cardiac and autoimmune diseases, as well as cancer.

Research carried out in the area of psychosomatics over the past 20 years shows a wealth of material and development. As mentioned above, there is no theoretical body to support such research, although the vast majority of the findings reveal highly significant data.

Evidence of a psychophysiological intersection is accumulating, which, according to Myers and Benson (1992), may be divided into three different levels. The first involves the countless correlations between psychological factors and physiological effects, and research that seeks to establish a relation between typology and a disease. It also includes observations of the relaxation response resulting from specific patterns of thought, which gives rise to physiological alterations such as diminution of oxygen consumption, elimination of carbon dioxide and changes in blood pressure, and how the presence of a person to assist before and during childbirth greatly diminishes the amount of time between admission and delivery, as well as the incidence of perinatal problems.

One of the most interesting phenomena at this level of research is the placebo effect. Regarded merely as part of an experimental design to test a new drug, the placebo effect was, until recently, generally disregarded. Today, hundreds of studies involving the placebo effect are being developed, proving the action of psychic factors on the body (see the Appendix).

The second research level shows a correlation between a psychological event and a biomolecular effect. We know, for example, that the lymphocytes of spouses in mourning show a marked reduction in activity compared to control subjects.

A third area of growing research is at a cellular level. Rossi (1986), among others, has shown how intercommunication develops between the nervous, endocrinal, and immune systems. Immunological cells carry hormonal receptors and substances similar to the hormone originating in the immunological cells. This type of research is beginning to show some possible paths to psychophysiological interaction at the organic level.

This chapter will concentrate on research concerning heart disease, rheumatoid arthritis and cancer, which are found within the first level, and will include some references to research in the second level. This review will by no means be exhaustive (the field is developing into a highly active sector); rather, the studies cited here are those that best substantiate, even indirectly, the analytical point of view.

Heart diseases and psychological factors

Friedman and Rosenman (1974), in describing the neurogenetic factors in the pathogeny of cardiac coronary disease, opened up fertile ground for research, which today probably constitutes the area of greatest investigative activity. Studying cardiac patients, they reported a multidimensional pattern of behavior characterized by:

1   driven behavior oriented to attaining goals
2   excessive involvement with one's job
3   an exaggerated sense of urgency
4   aggressive behavior

5 competitive behavior
6 impatience
7 vigorous linguistic and motor activity.

According to these authors, this combination of behaviors forms a personality trait they described as Type A, which has a high correlation with cardiac disease. Some authors even indicate that Type A men have a significantly higher excretion of testosterone glucuronide, which may represent a mechanism for the elevated incidence of coronary heart disease (CHD) in Type A men (Zumoff *et al.*, 1984). Several subsequent studies applied personality tests such as the Multiple Multiphase Personality Inventory (MMPI) and the Cook-Medley Hostility Scale (CMHS), and a structured interview was developed to differentiate cardiac patients from the normal population. As the studies were improved, however, one single trait was in evidence – hostility – that, as we shall see, includes some of these behaviors up to a certain point.

Hostility and anger

Research by Dembroski *et al.* (1985), Costa *et al.* (1987), Siegman *et al.* (1987) and Hecker *et al.* (1988) on the psychological factor of risk in CHD points to an antagonistic hostility trait defined as "a style of disagreeable and/or non-cooperative interpersonal interaction, that includes expressions of arrogance, argument, a sharp demeanor, and bad humor." Among individuals displaying a high level of this trait, for example, a greater difficulty in recovering from stress was discovered, along with a tendency for a considerable increase in blood pressure.

Other studies showed that people with either a high or a low degree of hostility present differences in cardiovascular reactivity during episodes of great interpersonal conflict. Suarez and Williams (1990) showed that very hostile men have a tendency to greater systolic pressure during episodes of great emotional conflict because they react rapidly with irritation and anger. Other results also indicate that anger and irritation lead to major changes in cardiovascular parameters, primarily in individuals with a high degree of hostility. In studies by Williams *et al.* (1991), Chesney *et al.* (1990), and Van Egeren and Sparrow (1990), there is evidence to suggest a significant link between frequency of anger and CHD. Hostile individuals that are involved in interpersonal conflict would be at greater risk than those who live in less challenging environments, conclude the authors. Results are more valid for men in the 35 to 55 year age group (Engebretson and Matthews, 1992).

In a study conducted over a period of 35 years by Harvard University, 126 university students were examined to determine the predictive value of previously studied psychophysiological standards in response to experimentation with stress in a laboratory. The most reliable variable in terms of an increase in susceptibility to CHD was "high anxiety", defined here as resulting from hostile impulses projected on others. Also significant were inter-punitive and extra-punitive expressions, associated with diffuse guilt (Russek *et al.*, 1990).

For 25 years, researchers Almada *et al.* (1991) studied 1,871 middle-aged male employees from the Western Electric Company, using MMPI. The only trait with a positive correlation with death by heart disease was that of cynicism, here described as chronic antagonism, stubbornness, and a rude and vengeful nature. Studies by Jamner *et al.* (1991) and Pope and Smith (1991) also show that men who are chronically hostile and more defensive present greater cardiovascular and neurohormonal reactivity, which, in turn, may initiate or worsen cardiovascular disease. Other studies such as Jorgensen *et al.* (2001) and Niaura *et al.* (2002) support this finding. Both found that hostility, alone or combined with high social defensiveness, is related to the development of coronary artery disease.

It is possible that hostility, characterized by cynical and denigrating cognitions, may serve to increase CHD risk by increasing the expectation that events will require an anger response. This would likely increase exposure of the subject to an anger-generated CHD risk. Accordingly, research that investigates the relation of anger to incidence of heart disease shows that both "anger out" (the likelihood of anger being expressed toward someone else during an extreme anger episode) and "suppressed anger" (the likelihood of anger being repressed or not expressed during an extreme anger episode) were positive predictive factors in the incidence of ischemic heart disease (Gallacher *et al.*, 1999). Along these lines, a study carried out in South Australia by Atchison and Condon (1993) indicated that the psychological factor that best predicted CHD was quicker experience of anger with greater verbal expression. Another interesting observation, made by Siegman *et al.* (2000), indicated that while full-blown outward expression of anger and dominance are risk factors for CHD in men, the more subtle expressions of antagonism (indirect challenge) are risk factors for CHD in women.

Clearly, it seems that hostility and anger are both closely related to the incidence of CHD, with the former now considered as a predictor of increased risk of myocardial infarction and death. These results have been observed in both genders (Lahad *et al.*, 1997; Chaput *et al.*, 2002) and in different cultures such as Denmark (Barefoot *et al.*, 1995), and Mexico (Gloria *et al.*, 1996), leading us to confirm the hypothesis that these phenomena are of a psychological nature, independent of cultural environment characteristics. In the Netherlands, for instance, Meesters and Smulders (1994) investigated patients with a first myocardial infarction who were later compared with a neighborhood control group. Their results indicate that hostility only constitutes a risk indicator for a first myocardial infarction in men who are younger than 50 years of age.

We may conclude that converging evidence from studies using different instruments suggests that hostility is the only predisposing component for a Type A behavior standard.

This type of study led to the development of techniques for behavior modification, the basic objective of which was to control or eliminate all manifestations of hostility through reinforcement and punishment, breathing exercises, and increased self-esteem (Ulmer and Friedman, 1984). Although these techniques may have some effect, the great problem is that dealing only with the symptom of concrete polarity makes the patient vulnerable to the unconscious dynamism that is synchronized with this behavior. The techniques control the behavior and disease, but do not promote the cure.

We might view the trait of "hostility" as just one aspect of the persona that acts defensively, leading to unilateral development of the conscience. The fact that these persons have an aggressive and hostile relation with the environment may only be the best expression of a specific complex and, as such, we should operate within this framework so that a cure may be found.

Depression and anxiety

There is cumulative evidence that other negative emotions such as depression and anxiety may precede the onset of acute coronary syndromes and influence the course of such diseases after their appearance (Appels, 1997; King, 1997; Kaufmann *et al.*, 1999; Williams *et al.*, 2002; Wulsin and Singal, 2003).

For example, Frasure-Smith *et al.* (1999) showed that depression in hospital after myocardial infarction is a significant predictor of one-year cardiac mortality for both women and men, and its impact is largely independent of other post-myocardial infarction risks. Lespérance *et al.* (1996) state that 40 per cent of those having a prior history of depression died within 12 months, whereas only 10 per cent of the patients who were experiencing their first episode of depression subsequently suffered this fate. It seems that depression not only poses a considerable risk for cardiac mortality and morbidity in patients with CHD, but has also been found to influence more general indicators of distress, disability, and quality of life (Sirois and Burg, 2003).

In a comparison of depression and anxiety, Strik *et al.* (2003) reported that while both are associated with cardiac events, anxiety alone was considered an independent predictor of cardiac events and increased healthcare consumption. The authors suggest that there may be more direct links between emotional states and the functioning of the parasympathetic nervous system, the immune system and heart rate variability. Decreased heart rate variability, seen as a lack of ability to respond by physiological variability and complexity, makes the individual physiologically rigid and, therefore, more vulnerable. This phenomenon was also observed by Horsten *et al.* (1999), who found that heart rate variability is lower in persons who are socially isolated and unable to relieve anger by talking to others.

It is highly likely that here we are seeing the activation of a complex, which, in addition to provoking the abovementioned physiological changes, simultaneously reveals defensive attitudes such as anxiety, heightened displays of anger, and social isolation.

Social support

In recent years we have also witnessed a growing interest in the impact of social support or social bonds on CHD (Cohen and Syme, 1985; Cohen, 1990). The line of research that helps to clarify this point has tried to establish a relationship between social support, job strain and cardiovascular reactivity. It essentially leads us to conclude that when the individual has emotional support, the probability of myocardial infarction occurrence is smaller when facing stressful situations (Gerin *et al.*, 1992).

Social support seems to offer stability that protects the individual in moments of transition and stress. Gore (1978) studied 110 men who lost their jobs when a factory closed down. He discovered that those who received strong support from their wives, relatives or friends had fewer heart problems than those who were isolated. Kamarck *et al.* (1990) proved that even in laboratory situations, subjects who were alone showed greater heart rate reactivity than those who were accompanied during a stressful situation. The presence of a friend had a calming effect on cardiac activity.

A study in Sweden conducted over ten years examined the significance of psychosocial risk in 150 Swedish men, concluding that the more precise independent predictor of mortality was the absence of social support, encountered mainly in Type A individuals (Orth-Gomér and Undén 1990). Probably owing to attitudes and hostile behaviors, this type rejects, is rejected, and has few or no loving relationships.

Another source of information in this respect comes from statistics indicating that susceptibility to disease is two or three times greater among single, separated, divorced, or widowed persons (Lynch, 1977, 1985). Matthews and Gump (2002) found that marital break-up increases the risk of post-trial mortality in men, while Gallo *et al.* (2003) proved that marriage appears to confer health benefits on women, but only when marital satisfaction is high. According to Orth-Gomér *et al.* (2001), marital (not work) stress offers a poor prognosis for women aged 30 to 65 with CHD, although after a population-based control study with women (Wamala *et al.*, 2000, 2001), it seems that cumulative exposure to socio-economic disadvantage also results in greater likelihood of CHD risk.

The discovery of Type A thus stimulated considerable research and established a relation between psychological events and the heart. Accordingly, we can add that behavior and psychosocial factors are demonstrably related to CHD. While we may label this as a "coronary-prone behavior", it does not represent a personality pattern such as supposed in the studies of Type A.

Although prolific and abundant, the literature that reveals the link among psychosocial factors, social bonds and cardiovascular risk does not clarify the mechanisms that produce it. These studies seemingly reveal and identify the phenomenon, but do not explain it. The mechanisms that explain such a relation remain unexplored. The reason that widowers and solitary and hostile individuals show a greater probability of developing CHD remains unknown.

Another question arises when we evaluate these studies: why, under the same stressful conditions, does a hostile individual have a greater probability of becoming ill than a non-hostile person?

We must try to understand how lack of social support can translate into myocardial infarction and, conversely, a loving, non-hostile attitude into a healthy heart. This will require studies focusing more on the psychic complex mechanisms than dwelling exclusively on social and conscious behavior.

At this point we can suppose that the onset of a complex can trigger the frequent psychological perception of threatening social phenomena, and, as a consequence, a reaction of anger, hostility or anxiety, which can be translated into a constricted artery or change in heart rate, for example.

Rheumatoid arthritis and psychological factors

An immune system that is functioning in a hyperactive mode may not be able to distinguish between the cells of the body and those that are foreign to it. The body will begin to attack itself and thus give rise to autoimmune diseases such as rheumatoid arthritis (RA) and cancer (Solomon, 1990).

In recent years, a growing number of studies and research findings have shown the possibility that mental events may have an effect on the immune system and its dysfunctions. In the following paragraphs, we shall focus on the studies that pertain most closely to our inquiry.

Patterns of obsessive behavior

Although the relation between RA and specific personality traits has not been shown in the scientific literature, Solomon (1981) and Moos (1964) observed that subjects with autoimmune diseases tend to be quiet, introverted, trustworthy, consenting, restricted in expressing emotions, rigid, conformist, highly active, and self-sacrificing. The observation that these characteristics are more common in women has been supported not only in my own clinical practice but also through several studies. According to a report produced by Symmons et al. (2000) for the World Health Organization – Statistical Information System (WHOSIS), women are almost twice as likely as men to be affected by this disease. More recently, an epidemiological study by Doran et al. (2002) observed the incidence of RA in a cohort group of 609 patients in Rochester, Minnesota, of which 73.1 per cent were women.

An interesting study in this area is that of Cabral *et al.* (1988), who observed an obsessive and hyperactive relation of women with RA towards work, primarily when working at home. This study on 59 women patients between the ages of 18 and 55 showed that work in the life of an arthritis patient represents an attempted flight from emotional conflict. This hyperactivity would be the product of an obsessive personality characterized by being organized, methodical, and rigid in conduct and duties. The authors interpret these data as a reaction to the low degree of worth attributed to housework. This conclusion was supported by research carried out by Marcenaro *et al.* (1999), who observed that obsessive-compulsive personality disorder was present in 40 per cent of their sample.

We may speculate that this result is not due to possible hormonal or genetic factors alone, but also to a feminine pattern of typecast victimization. This leads to the image of a woman with great creative potential, but whose daily activities are restricted to domestic chores or repetitive, monotonous jobs. This unrealized potential and its underlying energy will need to find a means of expression. The frustration of not finding a creative outlet for this energy may result in an obsessive-compulsive behavior, hence the exaggerated importance given to housework. On the other hand, it is likely that women who are able to develop a career or any meaningful creative activity may feel that they are more in control of their lives, as opposed to women who are limited to the execution of constant and repetitive tasks for their family members or demanding bosses.

The effect of employment pattern on health among women diagnosed with RA was also observed by Reisine *et al.* (1998), who found that employed women had better health status than those who were unemployed. They also noticed that those who had lost their jobs displayed the worst health of all. The authors state that employment has a protective health effect at the onset of a disease, and also a positive effect on pain relief, psychological distress and physical disability.

Stress

On the other hand, countless studies show that this disease seems to appear following a severe, stressful situation such as the loss of a loved one, or a switch from an established standard of living (Anderson *et al.*, 1985). In the abovementioned study of Marcenaro *et al.* (1999), the authors found that macro and micro stressful events preceded the onset of RA in 86 per cent of the subjects. They also found a correlation between stressful events and the outbreak of the disease in 60 per cent of the cases.

A study by Latman and Walls (1996) placed patients diagnosed with definite RA against patients with osteoarthritis, and found that the former exhibited more stress at the onset of the disease than the latter. Zautra *et al.* (1999) and Zautra and Smith (2001) carried out a series of studies proving that depression might be related to elevations in pain, whereas stressful life events are positively related to RA flare-ups, in the sense that interpersonal stressors were predictive of increases in disease activity.

One study seems to be less conclusive in terms of the hypothesis that exposure to stressful events and adverse experiences in childhood may play a significant role in the etiology of RA. Carette *et al.* (2000) conducted a retrospective study seeking to investigate whether early life events among a group of 116 subjects had any correlation with the development of RA. The authors noticed that termination of pregnancy was the only specific event individually associated with a higher risk of developing RA.

Until now, most of the research on this disease has employed intervention methods whereby the psychological treatment is evaluated in terms of immunological function. These interventions involved use of cognitive and behavioral techniques and focused on stress control.

Bradley *et al.* (1987) carried out an extensive study testing different types of treatment, and concluded that cognitive intervention with biofeedback and relaxation was effectively able to diminish levels of the rheumatoid factor and, consequently, inflammation of the joints. More recently, Sharpe *et al.* (2001, 2003) conducted a study on 53 patients with less than a two-year history of RA. All patients had received routine medical treatment, but 50 per cent of these also received eight weeks of cognitive and behavioral intervention. The authors reported improvements in both the depression index and joint functions of these patients, as well as a transient reduction in their C-reactive protein levels. Although these improvements were not maintained at six months' follow-up, as reported by the researchers, we may consider this information as important evidence that psychotherapy does have an effect on the physiological functioning of human beings. This temporary effect was probably due to the use of cognitive–behavioral techniques, which tap only the symptoms and do not promote deep psychological transformations.

On the other hand, when 15 patients were submitted to analytical insight therapy for 60–90 minutes each week over an average period of 3.3 years, six showed a major and continuous improvement in both their physical and their psychic state throughout a lengthy period after therapy. The other patients showed similar improvements after a longer period of therapy, but the authors noticed that the course of their disease became more variable after deeper emotional focus had been touched (Lindberg *et al.*, 1996).

Therefore, we may conclude that although the study of the influence of psychological factors on RA began fairly recently, one characteristic has been clear in rheumatic disease: it is more frequent in women, and in those with compulsive hyperactivity and obsessive rigidity regarding work. Stressful situations appear to bring about both the onset and aggravation of symptoms. It seems that those women who are victimized by monotonous, repetitive activities that offer few outlets for creativity are trapped in a complex that impedes behavioral change. In this case, the best expressive means in the organic polarity for this complex would be a gradual stopping of the movements, which symbolizes a psychic slowdown and acts as a compensatory mechanism, obliging patients to stop their aimless and compulsive hyperactivity. Studies conducted among a group of men could clarify whether this is a gender-specific pattern.

Cancer and psychological factors

Over the past few years, numerous researchers have tried to establish links between cancer and psychological variables. Due to the complexity of the variables involved, the results have been inconclusive. Critiques of the methodology employed have been one of the predominant factors in the analysis of the results and in the more positive use of the data.

As we will see, in getting a significant number of subjects for application of the statistics, the epidemiological studies fail to understand the psychodynamics involved. On the other hand, more detailed studies, which do not allow a quantitative analysis due to a smaller number of subjects, have had their validity questioned.

The following paragraphs highlight those studies that have investigated the behavioral variables most relevant to our inquiry.

Emotional repression

There have been countless suggestions in the literature that expressions of anger or, more precisely, the degree of emotional expression of a patient, have a bearing on the onset and progress of cancer. Reports of descriptive cases date from the 1950s, with a lower survival rate observed in depressed, resigned patients than in patients who are better able to express negative emotions such as anger.

Greer and Morris (1975) discovered that women diagnosed with malignant tumors in the breast experienced greater difficulty in expressing anger than those whose biopsy showed a benign tumor. Derogatis et al. (1979) reported that cancer patients regarded by the hospital staff as less cooperative lived significantly longer. These data contribute to another study by Greer et al. (1979), where breast cancer patients with "a fighting spirit" lived longer than those who showed a lack of hope and had a lack of support. Hislop et al. (1987) and Goldstein and Antoni (1989) found similar results among patients with breast cancer.

Some authors have sought a personality trait that might explain this "fighting spirit". Dattore et al. (1980), for example, used MMPI to test the hypothesis of a cancer-prone personality in a group of 3,000 US Army veterans from 1969 to 1978. Of this group, 75 men developed cancer. Compared with the control group, the researchers found that those with cancer had greater repressive tendencies.

Temoshok et al. (1985) put together the "expressive versus repressive" variables in terms of a Type C behavior standard. Temoshok and Dreher (1992) defined Type C as a cooperative, non-assertive patient that suppresses negative emotions, particularly anger, and that submits easily to external authority. As we can see, this standard Type C behavior is in contrast to Type A behavior. The authors carried out an extensive investigation on the relationship between Type C and the thickness and depth of the melanoma tumor. They found a significant correlation between the measurements of the tumor and Type C, particularly in patients under the age of 55.

Shaffer et al. (1987) conducted a study with 1,337 male medical students at Johns Hopkins Medical School, using 14 personality measures. Subjects were followed over a 30-year period to determine the cumulative survival rate (proportion of subjects remaining free of cancer) in each group. Statistically significant group differences in the survival rate were found, with the group characterized as outward and emotionally expressive having the most favorable results (less than 1 per cent developing cancer). The group characterized as "loners", who may well have suppressed their emotions, had the poorest results, and were 16 times as likely to develop cancer as the outward, emotionally expressive group.

The importance of expressing emotions to maintain health has been confirmed by some other studies. Faragher and Cooper (1990), for example, discovered that of 2,163 women who had undergone a breast cancer biopsy, the 171 diagnosed with malignant cancer tended to suppress their feelings and maintain few interpersonal relationships outside of the home or workplace, in comparison to the group of 1,110 women whose cancer was diagnosed as benign. Bleiker *et al.* (1996) investigated personality factors among 9,705 women in Holland who underwent a mammography during 1989–1990. After six years of monitoring these women, the researchers reported a weak association between a high score on the anti-emotionality scale and the development of breast cancer.

Tijhuis *et al.* (2000) investigated the relation between emotional control and the development of cancer in a study group of 590 men over a ten-year period, using the Courtauld Emotional Control Scale (CECS). Based on results showing 119 cases where cancer appeared, and 71 deaths linked to cancer, researchers discovered that the intermediate control of depression (a tendency to suppress the expression of one's depressive states) was related to cancer incidence, while both intermediate and high controls of depression were linked to cancer-related deaths. A recent meta-analysis has found that emotional repressiveness is a predictor of cancer incidence (McKenna *et al.*, 1999).

Studies that show what happens when individuals actively repress their emotional expression could explain the above results. Pennebaker *et al.* (1989) showed that these individuals displayed an increase of excitation in certain autonomous channels, such as in the electrical conduction of the skin. The authors observed that if an inhibitory process is maintained over a long period, it serves as a cumulative long-term stressor, augmenting the probability of falling ill. One particularly insidious form occurs when individuals experience a traumatic event and are incapable of sharing it with others. For example, studies show that individuals that suffered traumatic sexual experiences as children show greater probability of having later health problems if they do not discuss their experiences with others (Pennebaker and Susman, 1988). Also, those whose wives committed suicide or died in accidents were healthier one year subsequent to the death if they shared the event often enough (Pennebaker and O'Heeron, 1984). In two other studies (Pennebaker *et al.*, 1988), university students classified as "most revealing" showed a drop in the level of skin electrical conduction while they told of their very traumatic experiences. Over the long term, those revealing traumatic experiences showed a reduction in number of visits to the local health center up to four months following the study, and an increase in immunological functions up to six months after the experience. Studies with survivors of Nazi concentration camps reporting on their traumatic experiences showed that those who were less inhibited while reporting, measured by the drop in level of electrical conduction of the skin, were in better health than those who were less revealing (Pennebaker *et al.*, 1989).

All of these experiments support the results obtained by C.G. Jung during his association tests conducted at the beginning of the twentieth century. At the same time, they supply an important support for therapeutic activity by reinforcing the importance of reporting traumatic experiences and the expressiveness of emotions associated with them.

Severe life events and stress

Hundreds of studies in recent years have investigated the relation between stress, depression, and immunological function. Although we will not delve deeper into the subject at this time, we will include some of the data drawn from psychoneuroimmunology.

It would seem that the immune system reacts in a different way when exposed to acute or chronic stressors.

Some interesting studies on acute stress (that which is associated with a single event) have been completed with university students during exam time. Kiecolt-Glaser *et al.* (1984, 1986) carried out a series of studies to investigate a variety of immunological changes resulting from stress over school examinations. The results showed significant alterations in the immune systems of the students. Naliboff *et al.* (1991) subjected healthy individuals to a stressful situation in a laboratory, and found that the response to a threatening situation is an increase in the production of NK cells ("natural killers") and of lymphocytes, as if the body were preparing itself for a reaction of fight or flight. Esterling *et al.* (1990) found similar results with individuals who had to write down or who had to remember and to tell an intense emotional experience (Knapp, 1980; Knapp *et al.*, 1992).

When facing a situation of acute stress, the body reacts by activating its immune system, in the sense that it protects itself against an invasion. Diseases, however, do not necessarily follow these changes. The data show that great variations in immunological activity are possible without the onset of a disease.

During events of chronic stress, however, the reaction seems to be different. Prolonged unemployment, depression, and mourning are the chronic stressors that have been most studied. All seem to produce a lowering in lymphocyte response, with cases of prolonged immunosuppression (O'Leary, 1990). Sephton and Spiegel (2003), in their review of the neuroendocrine–immune pathway from stress to cancer, discuss the emerging data in the literature, which show that circadian regulation may also be an important prerequisite for the maintenance of host defenses against cancer. Stress-related circadian disruption, often present in states of chronic stress, may have negative implications for cancer prognosis.

Studies on stress related to mourning for a loved one, as well as the break-up of a relationship, have frequently associated it with the onset of malignant tumors. Autoimmune diseases usually become apparent after a person undergoes severe psychological stress that has totally changed his or her lifestyle (Solomon, 1990).

Temoshok (1985) discovered that melanoma patients classified as under great psychosocial stress were subject to more rapid progress of the disease, while Ramirez et al. (1989) reported that severe stress had a marked influence on the risk of a breast cancer relapse. Schleifer et al. (1983) tested the immune system in men whose wives were dying of breast cancer. They discovered that in the two months subsequent to their wives' deaths, the immune systems of the husbands were significantly depressed, but that they returned to normal from four to 14 months later. This discovery seems to be associated with the capacity to express pain; that is, those who wept in mourning recovered more rapidly than those who repressed it. These findings match those of Pennebaker and O'Heeron (1984) and Pennebaker et al. (1988), confirming that there is a relation between the inability to demonstrate suffering and concomitant suppression of the immunity. This may explain why there is an increased cancer risk among persons in mourning (Maddison and Viola, 1968; Solomon, 1990).

Geyer (1991, 1993) examined women aged 25–60 who had undergone a biopsy for breast cancer. Of these, 33 were diagnosed with a malignant tumor while 59 had a benign tumor. The conclusion was that the most severe life events – those associated with loss – were more common in the cancer group. Among this group, severe events were four times higher based on the scale used in relation to the control group. Serious, chronic difficulties were also more frequent in the group with cancer.

Kvikstad *et al.* (1994) conducted a study on the possibility of cancer risk increasing after the death of a spouse or divorce in a group of more than 600,000 Norwegian women born between 1935 and 1954. Of these, 4,491 developed breast cancer. The statistically adjusted results showed no clear evidence that the death of a husband or divorce had any bearing on increased cancer risk for these women. A similar study conducted in England (Jones *et al.*, 1984), showed little evidence for an increase in reported cases of cancer after the death of a spouse, and just a small increase in the number of deaths caused by cancer. Kvikstad and Vatten (1996) also observed that the risk of, and survival of, cancer were no different among women who had experienced the death of a child as compared to women without this experience.

Different results, however, were obtained by Levav *et al.* (2000), who investigated 6,284 Israeli Jews who had lost a son or daughter in the Yom Kippur War or in an accident between 1970 and 1977. The scientists reported a greater incidence of lymphatic and hematopoietic cancer, and melanoma, among those who lost a child than in the Israeli population as a whole. Also, the risk of respiratory tract cancer was greater among the former group. The survival study showed that the risk of death was increased by bereavement if the cancer had been diagnosed before the loss, but not after. Martikainen and Valkonen (1996) examined excess mortality among Finns after the death of a spouse and found a moderate (20–35 per cent) increase in the incidence of lung cancer, supporting the hypothesis that the loss of social support or the inability to cope may increase the probability of cancer.

The apparent contradictions between the results of these studies arise from the great difficulty of studying the mourning process. These studies did not consider the means by which these individuals handled the mourning, including religiousness and other variables. Furthermore, expressiveness and/or repression of pain would certainly have different internal repercussions for these people. Accordingly, stress-related studies ought to consider the emotional expressiveness and meaning attributed to the event, regardless of its origin.

On the other hand, studies that seek to measure the effects of

acute stress on the onset of cancer have encountered great methodological difficulties because the data for onset of malignancy is
inconclusive, and it is almost impossible to know whether a stressful
event preceded or followed the genesis of cancer.

Depression

An extensive epidemiological study of 2,020 employees of the Western
Electric Company (Shekelle *et al.*, 1981; Persky *et al.*, 1987), observed
that depressive symptoms in MMPI were linked to a doubling of the
risk of death by cancer 17 years later, and an incidence above normal
for the first ten years. A critical review of Shekelle's findings by
Bieliauskas and Garron (1982), however, showed that the grades in
depression reported as high were not within the pathological range.
More recent studies also failed to show such links. Hahn and Petitti
(1988) discovered no correlation between depression measured by
the MMPI and breast cancer in 8,932 women during 14 years of
observation. A ten-year study by Zonderman *et al.* (1989) also failed
to reveal significant depressive symptoms that might predict mortality by cancer. A more recent study, however (Irwin *et al.*, 1992),
showed that in depressed individuals, activity in the immune system
is considerably reduced, such that reduction in NK lymphocyte
activity seems to be more reproducible (cytotoxic activity of this
lymphocyte is involved in recognizing and destroying cells, both
malignant and those infected by a virus).

Andersen *et al.* (1998) supported these findings in a study carried
out on a group of 116 breast cancer patients who were assessed after
receiving surgical treatment. The researchers reported that the stress
level of these patients was linked to lower cytotoxicity of the NK
cells and with lower lymphocyte proliferative responses.

Although depression may alter the functioning of the immune
system (as with stress), this does not mean that it will necessarily lead
to the development of cancer in all such patients.

In general, in examining depressive states, the majority of studies
fail through a lack of specification. Most investigators do not differentiate between the several depressive disorders, nor have they examined the depressions in terms of past history, duration, or treatment
effected. Thus, through these studies, we cannot know the extent to
which depressive states may or may not influence the onset of cancer,
as the comparison of the results of different means to measure
depression are problematical. The studies did not specify whether

the "depression" being measured referred to a trait, a state, or a depressive disease.

When chronic depression was studied, the results indicated a clear correlation with cancer. Penninx *et al.* (1998) examined 4,825 Americans over the age of 71 with diagnosed depression, based on the classification by the Center for Epidemiological Studies (CES-D). After adjustment for age, sex, race, disability, hospital admissions, alcohol intake, and smoking, it was found that the excess risk of cancer associated with chronic depression was consistent for most types of cancer and was not specific to cigarette smokers. The researchers concluded that when present for at least six years, depression was associated with a generally increased risk of cancer.

Jacobs and Bovasso (2000) conducted a study of 1,213 women in an attempt to establish a link between death of parents/chronic depression and the development of breast cancer. The women were first examined in 1980, and again in 1995. Within this period, 29 women were hospitalized with breast cancer and ten died from cancer-related causes. According to the researchers, the psychosocial variables that suggested an increased breast cancer risk were death of the mother during infancy and severe episodes of chronic depression. The scientists also pointed out that the causative factors of breast cancer occurred and grew over a period of 20 years or more, indicating that recent events did not appear to increase the risk of cancer.

It is possible that a number of diverse childhood experiences may be associated with both depression and cancer. For instance, Felitti *et al.* (1998) found that four or more such events were associated with a relative risk of depression and of contracting any cancer.

Gallo *et al.* (2000) spent 13 years studying a group of 2,017 adults from Baltimore, Maryland. The findings showed a link between major depression and the onset of breast cancer among the women.

In research by Loberiza *et al.* (2002), 193 patients receiving hematopoietic stem-cell transplants were monitored over 24 months and were asked to complete questionnaires beginning six months after the transplant. The study concluded that depression was predictive of early death for those patients that survived less than 12 months after the treatment.

Another factor that has been studied in relation to cancer is hopelessness, which is a facet of depression. A study by Everson *et al.* (1996) analysed desperation as a factor linked to death and to the incidence of myocardial infarction and cancer in a group of 2,428

Finnish men, using a scale that measures this factor. They found that moderate and high scores of hopelessness gave rise to more than a twofold increase in the risk of cancer-related death.

Spiegel, one of the leading researchers in the field, considers that while the literature on depression as a predictor of cancer incidence is mixed, chronic severe depression may be associated with elevated cancer risk (Spiegel and Giese-Davis, 2003). According to Spiegel (1996), depression not only complicates coping with cancer and adherence to medical treatment, but also affects aspects of endocrine and immune function that may affect resistance to tumor progression.

Conclusion

We cannot say, based on these studies, that a specific type of personality will have a greater probability of developing cancer or RA. What the examples illustrate is that the non-expression of a strong, negative emotion, stemming from mourning, relationship break-up or a traumatic situation, is a factor that predisposes an alteration in the functioning of the immune system, rendering the body more vulnerable to the development of malignant tumors.

Stress, in itself and whatever its nature, is an aggravating factor when there is no possibility of expressing the emotions associated with it. However, studies that seek to measure the effects of acute stress on the onset of cancer have encountered great methodological difficulties because the data regarding the onset of malignancy is inconclusive, making it almost impossible to know whether a stressful event preceded or followed the onset of cancer.

Some studies have established a link between the immune system and psychological events. However, as the great majority of these studies were conducted by doctors and psychologists with experimental, social and/or physiological leanings and employed the use of tests and questionnaires, they were confined to social and conscious behaviors. The issue of how mourning, suffering, or compulsive attitudes may "relate" to the immune system can only be answered by means of studies that go deeper into more complex psychological patterns.

If on one hand the study of a placebo shows how a concrete symbol may act on the body, then on the other hand historical studies support the psyche–body interrelation in different systems and situations. However, both study types lack a theoretical framework that will integrate the two. The absence of theoretical referential bases limits these findings to the circumstances described, without allowing a deeper and more coherent understanding of the phenomenon. Certainly, these data will make sense and be of greater use when they are interpreted in the light of a theory.

To respond to these issues, nine clinical cases will be presented. They will be analyzed and interpreted based on the analytical model, and the research described above will be used as a reference. The first three cases (Chapter 5) will be presented in more detail; the others (Chapter 6) will describe the core therapeutic work.

Chapter 5

The analytical model in organic diseases

> But the sickness is also a symbol, a representation of something going on within, a drama staged by the It, by means of which it announces what it could not say with the tongue.
>
> (Groddeck, 1949: 101)

The cases described herein were selected mainly for their psychosocial significance. Diseases both coronary and of the immunological system have been seen as diseases of our era, both in numerical terms and in terms of the enigma they represent. We may consider the work with these patients as a paradigm for each of the diseases presented herein.

The therapeutic cases were analyzed in accordance with analytical methodology. Owing to the extent and complexity of the clinical material, the most illuminating analytical moments were selected. When possible, reliable transcriptions were made of the patients' dialog annotated during sessions, as also of their dream material.

The names and some personal data of the patients were modified to avoid any possible identification.

The human grenade: when the heart explodes (heart disease)

The patient, a 57-year-old engineer and senior executive in a multinational corporation, was referred by his cardiologist after having suffered a myocardial infarction about three months previously.[1]

History

Arthur is an only child; he says he was always a model pupil, never caused trouble for anyone. He affirms that he always adapted quite well to the most varied situations and never suffered any trauma or conflict. He lives in harmony with his wife and three children, enjoys a comfortable lifestyle, and says nothing upsets him, apart from this recent illness. He has had no prior illness except those of childhood. Constantly traveling to difficult business engagements, he enjoys this activity because he "can prove how good [he is] at competing." About three months ago, he began to feel "some sharp pains in the chest," but went to the doctor only when the pectoral pain increased, whereupon he was hospitalized with a myocardial infarction. Thus he discovered that he suffers from arterial hypertension, the probable cause of the infarct. He takes medication to control his blood pressure. He was referred to analysis for resisting the doctor's recommendation of cutting back on his work pace and of changing his lifestyle. The patient took the suggestion that he make time for more leisure to mean that he should increase his sports activities. He took part in a sports tournament that aggravated the hypertension.

First clinical observations

The first impression of Arthur is of a well-dressed man, slim and elegant – a persona of the perfect, successful executive. He seems very ill at ease during the first interview and resistant to the idea of therapy, "seeing that I don't have a single problem; my doctor ordered it." He shows himself to be closed off by speaking rapidly of his work and the challenge it represents. He is proud of his past and of having achieved everything with "much struggle and courage," because his parents were of humble origins and poor. He does not understand the relationship between the infarct and any sort of psychological problem, but is willing to investigate in order to "eliminate this disturbance." What seems to most discomfort the patient is the loss of control over his body and needing others to take care of him. Therefore, initially he agrees to therapy with the idea of thus ridding himself as soon as possible of his "discomfort." Any description of Arthur fits perfectly into the personality Type A discovered by Friedman and Rosenman (1974): aggressive traits, always involved in a chronic and unceasing competitive struggle, suffering from hostility and hurry.

Evolution of the analysis

The therapy focuses initially on his work, to which he devotes about 14 hours a day, not including weekend work. Having reached the pinnacle of his career, he feels little motivation, for he does not encounter as many challenges as he would like. He is highly competitive, walks and speaks rapidly, using aggressive and hostile words about his employees and colleagues. He demands the maximum of them, as if they were always in a championship.

He has insomnia; he always wakes up at 4:00 a.m. and studies the company reports. At 7:00 a.m. he is already in the office. He says he has no friends because he has no time "for idle talk." Of his wife and children he demands discipline and that they complete their duties; in this he says he has been obeyed. Apparently he is not conscious of how they live or what they feel. He sets up relationships unilaterally, issuing orders without hearing the replies. Even his amorous and sexual life with his spouse is rule-bound and disciplined, "to not upset the mind."

The same attitude characterizes Arthur during analysis. After relating each incident, which he usually reads from the detailed account in his appointment calendar, he raises his head and asks anxiously, "How about that?," "What do you think?," or "What do you make of that?" Since I do not react according to his expectations, despite his "striving to the maximum to be the best patient you ever had," Arthur leaves the sessions frustrated at times and apparently annoyed by my "inefficiency." His appointment calendar acts as middleman in our relationship, for it is there that he notes the interpretations. Empathy is difficult to establish, because Arthur takes pains to avoid any emotional contact. He sits on the edge of the armchair as if he were ready to stand up, which he does precisely when the time allotted to the session is up.

To the fifth session, Arthur recounts the following dream:

> I went to a business meeting, but it was taking place in a kind of amusement park. In a shooting gallery I get a nasty shock when I see my youngest daughter held fast as the target in an arrow-shooting contest. The arrows just miss her, and I wake up screaming.

Associations: the youngest daughter, aged 11, is his favorite. She is the only person that he is able to kiss, because she is not afraid of him and approaches him more spontaneously than do the others. When he was 11, his maternal grandmother, who was quite affectionate, died. From then on, he became more obedient and rigid, because she was the only person who protected him from his strict and demanding father.

He was greatly afraid of his father, who was "most correct and honest," although distant and given to explosions. His mother passed all her time completing domestic tasks with "incomparable precision." She spoke little and never expressed her emotions. He learned from her how "vulgar" it is to express emotion. Both parents expected their son to be brilliant, at least, and did not accept any evidence of inferiority.

Interpretation: this dream led the patient to speak for the first time of his childhood and his parents. Through this dream, we can see the origin of his hyperactivity and of his inflexible attitudes (which, however, do not bother him). Arthur continued to think, "that's the right way." The only thing that really upset him was the threat to his daughter, which we understand as the threatened loss of his emotionality. His anima, still in the infantile stage, finds itself threatened by arrows in a work environment (business meeting). The conflict seems to be set up between logos (work) and eros (anima), between the formal and rigid persona and the infantile and maternal (grandmotherly) emotional side. The arrows may be the hostile and aggressive attitudes, which are normal in his daily life. They may kill what is most dear to him. We might amplify the dream here. In a mythological context, arrows in the heart would represent an acute (sharp?) amorous suffering of which the patient is absolutely unconscious. The arrows would correspond to the cardiac symptom he was feeling a few days before the infarction (stabbing in the heart). Needing to "be Mr Tough," he did not pay attention to the symptoms until they became worse, forcing him to lie down, something he didn't like to do (insomnia, state of "constantly alert").

The psyche, by forcing him to lie down, to incline, forced him to the clinic, making him face a conflict, the fruit of an infantile complex. Insofar as he was unconscious of that conflict, the concrete polarity moved into his body as an infarct, visible in the symbol of "arrows piercing the heart."

Other dreams of similar cast followed that one. We began to perceive that the repressed desire for love had imprisoned him in a cold and objective world. The more he tried to rid himself of love, the more threatened he became. Here we remember the myth of Shiva, the Hindu god of creation. Lost in his meditations and daydreams, Shiva cuts himself off from nature, thus not allowing it to reproduce and blossom. Only the arrows of the god Madana in Shiva's heart awaken him. And thus, in an act of love, Shiva unites with Existence, giving form and matter to his thoughts (Albrecht, 1979; Ramos, 1990).

During the eleventh session Arthur mentions that, despite the medicine he takes to control it, his blood pressure is dangerously high. So we work with his symptom using the technique of active imagination.

I request that he try, with eyes closed, to "see" what was happening inside his body and where had this high pressure started. After about 30 seconds Arthur relates the following image:

> There is a man running down narrow streets. They seem to be channels, everything is very red. I think they're my veins. This man is running a lot and has a grenade in his hand. He can't stop, he always has to flee. Were he to stop, the grenade would explode.

This image explains why Arthur constantly had to be on the run. If the outside pressure (pressing business) were to abate, the internal pressure would be unbearable. Now Arthur can see that he always needs to be fleeing, running. He does not know exactly what he fears, but he is afraid to stop. We realize that he fears the emotionality associated with the feminine. He was afraid of becoming less a man, of weakening and becoming less efficient. That's why he ran, out of fear. The man with the grenade in his fist was associated with the strict and "explosive" father who punished him (he now remembered) for the slightest imperfections. The analysis, by touching on this complex loaded with energy and emotionality, worsened the cardiac symptom, in a way. That is, by making him more conscious of the conflict, the analysis made his fear more conscious, increasing his blood pressure; without a doubt, a normal fight-or-flight reaction when confronted by any danger.

Therefore, medication or lifestyle changes would have brought only temporary relief to this patient. Actually, he would not have been able to change his lifestyle in any definitive way, because a complex much more strong and dangerous than heart disease threatened him. Had we not worked with him, any other treatment would have been in vain.

This ties in with the observation of cardiac patients themselves that, although they know precisely what to do, they cannot follow the doctor's recommendations. Nor could it be otherwise, for a symbol far greater than consciousness is present: the symbol of the wounded, injured heart, which needs to be integrated into consciousness to bring about a real transformation.

Behavioral techniques based on punishment to control Type A behavior, if applied to such a patient, only reinforce neurosis and increase blood pressure.

The technique used to deal with the "human grenade" was also active imagination. I now propose to the patient that he enter into a dialogue with the "human grenade" (HG):

A: What do you want? What are you doing?

HG: I'm here to explode you. To get rid of you.

A: But why?

HG: Because I am full of hate, much hate. I can't stand so much hate. I want more and to explode everything.

A: Hate of what?

HG: I'm afraid. Afraid he'll catch me. I've no time to talk. Get out of my way.

A: *(Anxious and panting)* Wait a minute. Talk with me.

HG: Can you prevent the consequences?

A: I think so; we're not alone.

HG: I'm tired, very tired. I want to stop, but don't know how.

A: What's frightening you?

HG: He is. He who demands everything of me, who forces me to be like him, ready to explode.

A: Father?

HG: He himself.

A: Are you my father?

HG: No, stupid; can't you see, you idiot? It's he and not I. I am the victim he tortures.

A: But where is he?

HG: You don't see, you idiot. At the door to your heart!

At this moment, showing obvious fatigue, the patient stops and, moved by his emotions, speaks of the fear he had of crossing his father and of his aggressive explosions. We might be able to understand the "human grenade" as an aspect of his shadow that emerged in daily life as contained hostility and uncontrollable competitive impulses. With such a shadow, the patient had to stay constantly vigilant, ready to flee or fight, as his organic symptom revealed.

In the following sessions, we worked using the active imagination technique with the images that emerged spontaneously: the father in the door to his heart; the injured, bleeding heart; physical fights with the father; the free and empty heart; his daughter embracing his heart; and finally the warm heart, beating slowly.

During this phase, the patient presented a few episodes of arrhythmia and peaks of blood pressure.

Last dream of the analysis (29th session):

> I was cruising in an enormous gilded boat down a long canal. The boat was moving harmoniously, following the water's movements. And, at the same time, the banks of the canal grew wider and narrower, helping the boat to pass.

Associations: Gilded boat, boat of the twilight of middle age, which brings a sensation of pleasure and peace such as he had never felt before. The canal that moved reminded him of the rhythmic movement of the vaginal canal during birth. And it was thus that he felt himself, being born.

Interpretation: Already given by his own associations. Any addition would be redundant or reductionism. This dream reveals the birth of a new consciousness and a new rhythm in his psychic life. The canals (veins and arteries) were now free to offer passage to a renewed ego (boat).

After this dream, three more sessions followed in which his process was reviewed and confirmed. The patient asked to halt analysis, which was granted. At the present moment, 17 months later, he remains without further analysis. We know from his doctor that he no longer presents any symptoms, with his blood pressure normal.

There were a total of 32 sessions, two sessions weekly of 50 minutes each.

Central symbol of the process

We might say that this was a brief analytic process, focused on an organic symptom and which led the patient into his process of individuation (see Figure 5.1). When approaching middle age, in the metanoia, the individuation process blocked by a neurosis that the patient with resistance refused to acknowledge emerged as a symbol

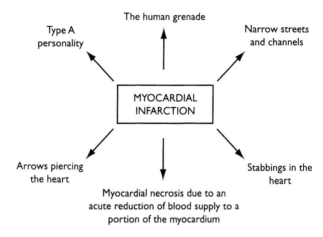

Figure 5.1 Case summary of "the human grenade" (myocardial infarction).

at the concrete, corporeal pole, forcing the patient to confront his complexes and correct his one-sided development. What might have been lived on the abstract plane had to be experienced synchronistically on the concrete plane, due to his lack of consciousness, in order to be integrated into his consciousness.

His becoming conscious of the parental complexes and the perception of the shadow as a hostile and destructive aspect, the "human grenade," were the core realizations in this process. From the moment when he became conscious of this shadow, his anima could be liberated, albeit in an infantile stage, and a more balanced and loving attitude could be developed.

The stoic: when joints flare up (rheumatoid arthritis)

Beth is a 49-year-old housewife who has been suffering from rheumatoid arthritis for ten years.[2] She sought treatment with psychotherapy because she felt very depressed and useless.

History

Beth is a married mother of four children, of ages ranging from 20 to 28 years. Her husband is in business and keeps his family on an average socio-economic level. She began to feel pain in her hands and knees around ten years ago, but did not get upset about it until the freedom of her movements diminished. She walks with a certain degree of difficulty and fatigues rapidly. The hand joints already suffer rather visibly from deformities. The joints of the wrists, elbows, knees, ankles, and toes have also been affected, but to a lesser extent. She notes that the symptoms worsen when she is tense and irritated. She has been treating the condition with medicine for six years without any improvement. She has tried acupuncture and homeopathy, also without noticeable effect. Occasionally she takes anti-inflammatories to relieve the pain.

First clinical observations

Beth seems intimidated and ill at ease. She extends a greeting by stretching out one hand and hastily withdrawing it, as if she were afraid she would not be greeted in return. Her touch is light and evasive. She sits down on the very edge of the armchair firmly holding on to her purse on her lap. She speaks in a low voice, looking down at the floor. Her appearance is frail. Her hair is bound in a tight bun, her clothes are stretched, and her white wrinkled hands convey the impression that she just emerged from a bath of chlorine. This impression is accentuated by the odor of chlorinated water emanating from her hands. She says she would never have imagined that some day she would require help, for she had always managed everything on her own. She works a great deal at home and at a church where she sews for the poor, so that she did not know how she was going to find time to take care of herself. She decided to go for treatment owing to the insistence of her youngest daughter, and there she was "at my orders."

Evolution of the analysis

Beth commences her first sessions with a description of her household duties, with much precision and in detail, to tell of all the care she devotes to her family. She says her form of expressing love is, for example, to butter the bread and have the coffee and milk ready in each one's cup so that they will not be late in the morning. Clothes washed and pressed, a clean, organized house, and delicious nutritious food are, according to the patient, her way of conveying her affection.

Although she can afford to pay for a maid or domestic help, she refuses to do so "because nobody else knows how they like it done."

Her obsession with cleanliness is such that she will only go to sleep after everyone else, so that there will be no print of a shoe on the polished flooring of her hallway. She says that to go on doing all of this, even in pain, is the best way to show, even further, her love for her family.

Her relationship with her husband is cold and distant. She feels very hurt because he does not comprehend this form of affection and insists on frequent sexual intercourse, even when she is ill or tired. This seems a formal relationship where the husband amuses himself with his friends while his wife cooks and takes care of the children. The children have become her refuge and her reason to avoid the husband. She associates the onset of "pins-and-needles" and of burning in her knees and hands with her youngest daughter's leaving home. At that time her life became more solitary.

During analysis, she started to associate her excessive work with a defense mechanism against the fear of being abandoned. She realized that she increased her workload to shut out the feeling of loss and solitude. However, she never complained or argued in order to avoid annoying anyone. Her basic attitude was one of subservience and modesty. She never spoke back, even when she was sure that she was right. She was horrified by conflicts and avoided them by "shutting up." In fact, permanent muscular constriction of the oral area could be observed, with "pursing" of the lips.

We began to talk more of her conflicts and resentment, of which she seemed to be gaining awareness for the first time. The patient, however, often fell silent, saying she had nothing more to tell. We gradually became aware that this mutism hid her fear that she might be annoying me with her complaints, and that I might consider her "ungrateful." Negative maternal transference was thus gradually established and, by degrees, the patient could perceive that she was reacting as though I were her repressive and critical mother, who, indeed, would not allow "whining and complaints."

The negative maternal complex of this patient had created a rigid personality structure with a weakened and split ego. Her desires, always considered "lesser things," were so repressed that they were inaccessible to the patient herself. Revealing her sentiments was at times accompanied by worsening pain. It was as if each repressed emotion corresponded to a contracted muscle, and the possibility of expressing it might be followed by punishment (as her mother used to punish her). The patient began to reveal deep sadness about her desires put aside, their place taken by the sense of duty (which guaranteed that she would be accepted), and spent innumerable sessions weeping copiously.

Beth began to realize that her masochistic and depressive structure had led her to sacrifice herself continually for others, to the point of dressing in old, mended clothes, much beneath her buying power, which would preclude "the danger of criticism for spending too much."

During this period, the patient brought the following dream:

> I am in an ugly street full of holes and gutted by the rains. There are two trucks loaded with cartons of eggs. They are trying to go uphill, but they are top heavy and skid downwards. The drivers are forcing the engines to such an extent that they are overheated, and there is threat of fire.
>
> (10th session)

Associations: The patient associates the steep slope with her parents' street where she was brought up. The torrents of water would be associated with her mania for cleanliness and her continual efforts washing down the back yard with a hosepipe. The trucks, laden, refer to her permanent feeling of body weight and difficulty in walking. She associates eggs with something new to be developed.

Interpretation: Through this dream, we were able to begin to perceive how her continuous efforts in "washing" were producing "holes" that impeded a normal flow of traffic. Although as a first dream we may observe a positive possibility for analytical development through the eggs, an excess of it also brings difficulties. Potential of such considerable weight, but unused for so many years, implies that there would have to be some loss for possible use of it. That is, some eggs would have to be set aside and the floor would have to be less clean so that the trucks would be able to reach their destination. The patient herself came to this conclusion, and we talked about how this might take place in her day-to-day life. To force an ascent with a full load under these conditions would mean the outbreak of fire, and at this time, the patient remembered a burning feeling in her joints. She realized that when she tried to force the "uphill drive" by trying to excess, the sensation of burning and pain in the joints was augmented.

On the other hand, to relinquish hold of her newly found wishes was no easy task. And to carry on, bitter and resentful, not having fulfilled them was also, seemingly, not the best way out.

The patient began to recollect how she used to enjoy music and dancing as a child, and how she had denied herself these pleasures because she felt awkward and stiff. It was as if all that was life and flexibility had been tied up and the patient, imprisoned in chains, was restricted to rigid and limited movements. Her self-sacrifice had only been halted by the illness, which had worsened in the past few years.

Until then, she had blindly obeyed all outside requests. Her altruism turned obsessive, and when she could not complete a given task she was possessed by a feeling of unbearable anxiety. She then realized that her body was defending her from further abuse because she had never said no.

Ziegler (1983) associates rheumatoid arthritis with the Stoic philosophy, in which patience, obedience and altruism played predominant roles. The Stoics, like the patient, belittled the body and subjected themselves to the most severe physical conditions with the idea of reaching a superior state. They were self-sufficient and avoided emotions, impulses, and desires.

Slowly we came to realize that the patient was not able to give up her stoicism, for this was the only form of power she exercised. Being above desire gave her a feeling of superiority, a sentiment that could not be substituted. Her limitless physical activity, although senseless and useless, afforded her a sensation of superiority. "Needs" were something inferior, belonging to less evolved beings.

Other dreams:

> I am on a motorcycle. I stretch the rear part and out comes a cover on which a woman and a girl sit. I set off at high speed. On the way, there are ever so many slats and boards. There is only one narrow curved passage along which I travel. I leave the two women. I take a car that a man is driving. He goes up a very steep slope of dark earth. He goes too high and falls, but the road goes on normally.
>
> A black car is going up a steep slope and boils midway. It almost goes on fire.
>
> (25th session)

Associations: The patient sees a motorcycle as a swift agile vehicle, but has never ridden on one. The two women are reminiscent of herself and her mother. The man is unknown, and the steep slope resembles that of the former dream. A black car resembles her father's old car back in the 1950s.

Interpretation: We may observe that analysis has liberated an enormous quantity of energy (imprisoned in the maternal complex), represented by a swift and flexible motorcycle. However, when she leaves the women and is being driven by a man, he forces his way up and the fall occurs. We began to realize that when her masculine side had taken over control, it had forced her into a stoic attitude, which led her to disaster.

The patient remembered that her mother only paid attention to her when she did her chores right, and the relationship with her father centered even more on her scholastic and domestic achievements. She had strived too much to be loved by him; he admired "objective," "thrifty," and "unemotional" women. She thereby assumes a paternal repression as to her femininity, an issue clearly evident in the following dream:

> I open an antique wardrobe. It is full of old men's jackets. These are male coats without the trousers.

Associations: Old jackets would be the father's jackets. There are no trousers because she feels she donned only the top part. "The top half, I am a woman. I have children to prove it when my husband complains I am not a woman."

Interpretation: These paternal jackets would be the armoring that the patient herself uses in her relationships. These are jackets that compel her to be distant and "objective." However, they are old, as an attitude that is already worn and close to consciousness. One part of her feminine identity was preserved in maternity.

In the 37th session, the patient reported in surprise that it was days since she had remembered her arthritis. Although it was winter, the pain had diminished considerably, to the extent that she had forgotten about her illness.

I proposed to work directly with the illness, once its regressive aspects became more conscious. The patient concurred.

I ask her to sit comfortably and concentrate, eyes closed, on the most painful joint. The patient says it's her knee. I ask her to concentrate on this point, trying to observe what is happening there. The patient states that it's a type of "distress" along with certain "soreness." "A weird soreness that gets better when I put my knees together." As she touches her knees together and then spreads them, she realizes that this is a defensive movement against an invasion – sexual invasion by her husband. At this point intense hatred for her husband surfaces, mixed with nausea and revulsion; sentiments she had never realized before.

She remembers countless times when she was indisposed or resentful of her husband, but nonetheless had sexual relations "because it was my wifely duty" and a form of "guaranteeing that he won't look for another woman."

We began to understand that the hardening of this joint was a defensive mechanism against movements imposed against her will. In reality, the arthritis in her knee was a defense that aimed at protecting her against this violation and, at the same time, the best way to express her Self, given the conflict between the wish for power (keep her husband) and eros (hate her husband). Restriction of movement protected the patient from a greater evil, continuing a hateful relationship.

She brings the following dreams to the next session:

> I see a leafy tree, but all dried up on the outside. I cling to a vine full of sap to grab two yellow fruits which are in the treetop.
> A friend's father welcomes me with affection, bestowing love on me.

Associations: "I myself, as the world sees me, am the tree. Dry, lifeless. But inside I have sap and can bear fruit, only it is still difficult to get to them." "I envy a friend who had a father who was always a companion to her and affectionate."

Interpretation: The patient begins to realize the dissociation between how she expresses herself and her inner world. She is surprised to realize that she has "sap," i.e. creative life within herself. At the same time we might say that there is an improvement in the paternal complex, which now appears in its positive polarity.

In the succeeding sessions, we continued working on the joints' symptoms, giving them voice. As will be seen in the account below of a session, anger is the predominant emotion that surfaces from the technique of active imagination.

42nd session: The patient, already more conscious of the tensions in her knees, proposes investigating the pain in her right wrist, which has particularly bothered her in the past few days. Eyes closed, she concentrates her attention on this point. She describes a heightening of the pain, as if there were a handcuff tightly securing her wrist. I ask her to imagine this handcuff tightening even more and then to try to "see" who is on the other side of it. The patient feels the heat rising, as if the handcuffs were scorching her skin, and "sees" her husband laughing, sadistically holding a key. The image of the husband is mixed with that of her father, and the patient weeps with anger, feeling herself powerless. Faced with the power of the two men, she could do nothing.

> I am a marionette tied at the wrists and ankles, which dances to the tune they play. I have no will of my own. I walk and jump incessantly at their will. No one protects me. I have to do as they command.

The patient emerges from her active imagination crying a great deal and gets up, wanting to leave before the end of the session. She feels her wrists and ankles are burning and complains that now it is much worse than it was before she began therapy.

I ask her to go back to active imagination and try to talk with her father/husband, which she does somewhat reluctantly. After a few seconds, the patient opens her eyes saying that it's useless to continue, that there's nothing to do. We stay this way, with this impotent feeling to which we refer later in other sessions and which was reinforced by the image she had had previously, upon falling asleep: "I was having trouble falling asleep. I breathe with difficulty. I see my wedding ring restricting my chest, keeping me from breathing more freely."

57th session: During active imagination, I propose to the patient that she concentrate on her body and the joint that calls out the most. The patient directs her attention to her atrophied fingers. She is hardly able to open them, so painful is any movement. There returns the sensation of handcuffs on her wrists and she realizes that she will have to use her fingers to get free of them. Neither her husband nor her father will come to her aid. She will have to do it alone. I realize that the patient is beginning, with great effort, to move the fingers of her right hand, as if she were opening a padlock on her left wrist. She repeats the motion with her left hand. Her motions are slow and apparently painful. She ends the effort smiling. She knows that she is not free yet, will have to repeat this movement again and again, which she does spontaneously at home, various times each day.

In the following sessions, Beth states that she is able to move her painful fingers for the first time in years. She feels that the sap of life is flowing toward the outer limbs and the dry tree is starting to come alive. She is already more able to reach out, and begins to fight with her husband and children.

I offer guidance that she should exercise at home with an image of this sap flowing throughout her body, centering on the regions more affected. After a few weeks, we could see a considerable improvement in the inflammation and the pain, principally in her knees, wrists, and fingers.

At the same time, her fights with her husband become more aggressive, and he refuses to go on paying for his wife's treatment, in retaliation to what he describes as a terrible worsening. Without any professional preparation whatsoever, the patient cannot find a job, and, after some sessions, treatment is suspended.

Beth returns once a month for one year, reporting on her battles with her husband and the new social position she has attained. She gets a job as saleswoman in a shop and changes in the way she dresses. Her appearance now is far more jovial and cheerful. She says she can "maneuver" her husband and does as she pleases. Although the rheumatoid arthritis has not gone away completely, she no longer feels pains and the inflammation emerges in her hands only when she is tired or stressed.

She understands that the illness may return if she detours from the "path of her Self," if she stops "obeying herself" and begins to "obey the others."

Central symbol of the process

We realize that the rheumatoid arthritis, from being a symbol, has changed to being a sign – a sign that advised her when she was exceeding a limit and losing her balance (see Figure 5.2).

There were 79 sessions, of 50 minutes each, over the course of two years.

Some of this patient's aspects correspond to the descriptions in the literature on patients with rheumatoid arthritis, i.e. she showed a rigid, complying, overactive, and self-sacrificing personality.

According to the patient, the triggering stress factor was loneliness aggravated by her youngest daughter leaving. However, as we were able to observe, the frustration and anxiety predated the daughter's departure, and there were dysfunctional signs long before that event.

Arthritis, as a symbol, is here associated with the parental complexes. Her compliance and subservient behavior were the

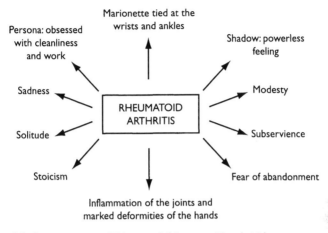

Figure 5.2 Case summary of "the stoic" (rheumatoid arthritis).

mechanisms used to protect her from the possibility of rejection, with false altruism used to defend against the anxiety of not being loved.

The illness, by stopping her movements, also stopped the continuation of her defensive, obsessive, and servile hyperactivity. If, on the one hand, repression of desire created a feeling of superiority, on the other hand it produced intense sorrow and resentments, which were accumulating in the joints.

By stopping, the organism rebelled against detouring away from normal development. Nodules of sorrow accumulated in the body, signaling the need for transformation. Paradoxically, this illness saved her from a worse evil: continuing to live without desires, unconnected with her Self. We might note that the inflamed joints revealed the "inflamed psyche," her silent revolt against the constant violation of her essence.

If the stiffness revealed, from one point of view, the stiffness of her psyche, from another it was the symbol by means of which the patient was able to retake control of her process and let the "sap flow once more."

The depressive: when cells revolt (cancer)

Cecilia is a 32-year-old teacher who seeks analysis because, after surgery to remove a melanoma,[3] she is very afraid of dying.

History

Cecilia is single and lives with her mother. About two months ago, the birthmark that she had on the left side of her right leg thickened and began to itch and bleed. She went to a doctor who diagnosed a melanoma, which was then removed. She states that she was very depressed for months before the cancer appeared, because she and her ex-fiancé had broken up about seven months previously. The plans for the wedding had already been made when he decided to go back to his former wife. Unable to accept these facts, she fell into despair, pursuing him at work and at home. During this time, there were days when she did not have the strength to go to work and stayed at home weeping. Subsequent to surgery she was somewhat more at peace and more resigned. She attributed the illness to her emotional suffering and death wish. The illness startled her, and she decided to react, although she still fell into profound states of depression and, at times, the idea of killing herself reappeared. She claims that "if I go on this way, I really will die," and "the disease will take over and there will be nothing to stay its course." She hopes that analysis will somehow help her to "feel better or to die more quickly and without pain."

First clinical observation

Cecilia seems older than her actual age. Her face marred by wrinkles, her graying hair and the sadness in her expression make her seem worn and bitter. She cries a good deal as she tells of the pain of separation, and is calmer only with the fantasy that "one day he will be sorry and come back once more." When she discovers that this is quite impossible, she falls into depression once more and cries.

Evolution of the analysis

Analysis in the first sessions consisted of taking in the patient's suffering. Her continuous desperate weeping prevented any analytic intervention. A psychiatric consultation was suggested for anti-depressive medication, which the patient refused. She said she could "hang on" and, on the other hand, she was sure that once she was in possession of the medication, she would not resist the temptation and would use it to kill herself.

The first analytic dream (fifth session) placed the process in a

positive perspective and, in part, reassured the analyst, who feared
that the patient would commit suicide:

> I was at sea with other people. I had to cross over to the other
> side to a beach that was in front of the beach where I was. The
> waves were extremely high, and in the sea there were some white
> animals that seemed like seaweed burning. I already had a burn
> on the back of my right hand. Where the waters from both
> beaches met, there was a great impact of water. But, I had to get
> over to the other side, and I kept trying. I knew that if I could
> traverse this stretch, it would be easy enough to reach the other
> beach. I made it. A girl came out of the water, naked, with me.
> There were a great number of mosquitoes. We went on as far
> as the road, and I asked for help. A car stopped, gave the girl a
> towel and we left in the car.

Associations: The sea gives a sensation of crossing. She has to under-
take a crossing: white dangerous animals threaten her and she recol-
lects that, as a child, she had suffered jellyfish burns while walking
barefoot on the beach. The father had, at this time, just left home
to live with another woman. A burn also makes her think of
melanoma.

Interpretation: As an initial dream, we may understand it as a
positive prognosis in the analytic process. The crossing is difficult;
however, the dreamer can make it. There are burns and bites from
primitive animals, but that can be overcome. That is, along the way
there will be painful situations, but results are positive in the sense
that from the sea there emerges a naked girl divested of her persona,
and both follow along the same way. Memories of the father are
painful and are associated with abandonment. It is probable that
there is a strong paternal complex associated with the shadow as an
abandoned little girl.

Cecilia always had several birthmarks distributed around her
body, which she associated with her father, as he had similar marks.
Upon removing the melanoma, she thought she was cutting a link to
her father, breaking a connection to him, and felt relief on the one
hand and great fear of losing him on the other.

Her parents' separation happened when the patient was 11 years
old. It was a very difficult event, because her mother did not accept
the separation and made "scandalous scenes" to get the father back.
Her mother never recovered, got depressed, acted as an abandoned

child, and created a series of difficulties for her daughter and for the younger brother. This brother lives abroad and for years has not been in touch with the family. From a very young age, he would be away from home and would spend more time at the house of friends. The patient would then feel responsible for the mother and feel guilty when she left her on her own.

She considers the period when she was with her fiancé (one year) the happiest in her life. He accepted her mother, and she even felt that the three might live together. She developed a series of fantasies as to how they would live and could not understand the reason for their breaking up, as they rarely quarreled. She attributed separation to pressure from her fiancé's ex-wife. However, later she realized that he really couldn't care less about her. To him, "it had been no more than a pastime and sexual attraction." It was at this time that she fell into depression.

The patient recounts numerous dreams that have a common pattern: accident, illness, and death.

> I was at home: my mother was in another room. I am very afraid of burglars. I had died, and they had only found my body two days later. At first, I thought it was suicide, but later they found an arm and a leg broken. But I still thought it was suicide, for I had been dead for two days and bones break very easily.
>
> They are digging a grave in the cemetery. They take away all the earth. I can see a coffin: it resembles a crate. In it is the body of a girl. In the tomb are two older corpses. They walk along with the coffin past one of these shelves with a corpse. They say it smells bad. I look on from without. A girl cousin of mine tampers with one of the coffins, and I can see the face. It is a skeleton of one of the corpses.
>
> An enormous crash. It's a collision of two trains that are moving backwards.
>
> (25th session)

Associations: The patient was much moved by these dreams and associated them with a feeling of solitude and loss. A cemetery is a place where she likes to go. "I should like to be able to get inside a tomb and go to sleep."

Following these associations, the patient was quiet. With lost gaze, she seemed unreachable for some moments. On her return, she said that she felt as if she were in this tomb and that there, although it was cold and malodorous, was where she wanted to be.

Interpretation: Although the patient was not yet in a state to absorb any deeper analysis, we could understand these dreams as a portrait of the trauma that the patient underwent when her love relationship ruptured. On the other hand, through analysis Cecilia began to discover past situations when she had probably already felt the same suffering, which left her lacking energy and depressed. The trains moving backwards and crashing might indicate conflictive regression: a catastrophic collision similar to the clash of the two seas in the previous dream, only now on a more conscious plane. The hypothesis that in this break she would be reliving abandonment by the father will soon be confirmed.

I ask Cecilia to try to recollect when she might have felt as if she were in a cold, malodorous place. She remembers sitting on the steps in the backyard of her house watching her father packing his suitcases into the car. She can say nothing. She would like to stop him, but she cannot move. The mother is making a "scene" and would like her daughter to do something about it. She feels cold and cannot move. All she would like is that her mother would stop talking. She would like to go to a place where it was quiet, without shouting. She does not want to go on talking. She feels pain where she had the surgery.

We begin to disinter the corpses. One of them is her father's. She had to be "hard." She could not fall into despair, as had her mother. She had always hidden her suffering, pretending that all was well to "cheer up" her mother. She had always been a model pupil and daughter, accepting all aggression without responding in kind, not touching on the subject of "father," and avoiding involvement in confused situations, in order not to make her mother even more "nervous." She rarely got together with her father, and on these occasions, fearful that he would not return, she tried also to talk only of "good things, to not irritate him."

We could see here that this patient possessed personality traits similar to those described in the literature as Type C. Loneliness, self-sacrifice, and resignation had been her defense. And her personality had been structured along these lines.

We worked thoroughly on these aspects, and anger began to emerge. She returned to the moment of her father's departure, using active imagination, and was able then to express all her emotions and resentments. In these moments she complained of pain in the region of the surgical scar, for which there was no medical reason.

We also began to realize the similarity between the situation experienced with her father and that with her ex-fiancé, with whom she clearly showed the wish to resolve what the child had not been able to do with the father.

On one hand, she was her father's daughter; the intellectual, a good student, and disciplined, who had abdicated from the more erotic aspect of life to devote herself to her profession. On the other, she was possessed by a negative identification with the mother. "She was horror-stricken" at resembling her, a "weak and dependent woman" and, nonetheless, in the case of her fiancé, she found that she had spoken much as had her mother.

The negative maternal complex had constellated in her difficulty in making female friends, in viewing all women as inferior to men and in her alienation from her own body. She took care of her body as a duty, rather than with pleasure. She kept it "clean, hygienic, and healthy" as an obligation.

Dreams

> I can see three black police dogs. A woman is holding them by the collar. They escape and attack me.
>
> I look through a window at ballet dancers going through their paces. They repeat the movements until they are perfect.
>
> (40th session)

Associations: "Fear of dogs, mainly of police dogs. I invariably have the sensation that they are going to attack me for no reason. They are angry. Something is going to break loose out of control. I cannot trust a woman. Ballet dancers are perfect, light. They must kill themselves before they attain perfection."

Interpretation: A liberation of anger has begun (that she sees in the dogs). She is afraid of losing control and hurting somebody (or herself?). A desire for perfection comes from a paternal complex. She has always tried to be "perfect" like he is, a perfect man. The ballerina is one who transcends perfection, who carries out her duties, even if for such she must repress her body and distort it to achieve "superior movements."

In another dream:

> A very important man is going somewhere, but does not want to

be seen. Then, there is a fleet of black cars. Three men are dressed the same way, and get into three parallel cars. One of them is the chief. This was one way to throw the others off the track. Many black cars follow along to protect him; however, the enemy filters through in disguise, in amongst the cars. All make their way to a tunnel, but the three cars are blocked. I tell somebody that there is no point in going on because the cars have been blocked.

(45th session)

Associations: "Black cars are Mafia cars. They are trying to protect the Big Boss. I don't know whether the enemy is the police or another rival group. A feeling that there is no way out. Danger. My father's car is black. It reminds me of the scene of the wedding of the daughter of the Mafia Big Boss in the film *The Godfather*. I find the women are submissive to the power of the men and have no way out."

Interpretation: The paternal complex in its negative polarity is manifest here as repressor and controller. Retaining power, he is not going to forfeit his daughter very easily. On the other hand, in the dream, this power is under threat. The conflict blocks a channel of energy (tunnel), but is closer to consciousness. How to tackle this power is the next question.

Another dream:

I am an Indian. They kill my boyfriend. I am about to drink water, and I find him dead in the tank. I am shocked. There is an enormous Indian beside me. I say I will bury him. I roam over the land. There is somebody with me. I say I want to bury him alone. I don't need the help of the people down below. Some domestic animals follow me. A duck and a sweet little donkey. I know the enormous Indian is going to carry my boyfriend so that I may bury him.

(47th session)

Associations: "Indian, a strong primitive man. I believe he was shot dead by the police. It's like the Wild West films. The Indians being shot by the army."

Interpretation: If we take the figure of the Indian to be the animus, his death by patriarchal power once again represents the imprisonment of the patient by the paternal complex. The positive aspect of this dream is the presence of other primitive forces (Indian and animals) that help her on her journey.

The patient feels blocked and bereft of energy. Absorbed as yet in pain, she cannot produce and work.

Dreams:

> My house is on fire. I watch from a distance. I am in a car with my mother. Everything is very dark: we are on the expressway. I have to stop the car because I cannot see a thing.
>
> The car battery has given out, so I will plug into the electricity.
>
> (49th session)

Associations: "It's exactly as I feel, devoid of strength, with no will. I don't know how to plug the car into the electricity."

Interpretation: The patient is depressed and perceives uncontrolled emotion (fire) destroying her life, and in the absence of her own energy, she tries to connect herself up to a social source (electricity network) that, nevertheless, depends on a connection and does not permit her to move very far. She comes to the conclusion that, at this time, this would be the best solution, i.e. to connect through to what society has to offer.

Dream:

> I am leaving the house to take my grandmother some place. I am in the car with my mother and another two girls. I sit in the back seat, and my grandmother sits in the driver's seat. I tell her it is impossible to drive like this. I show my mother that I cannot reach the steering wheel and the foot pedals. Then, with difficulty, my grandmother moves into the back, and I move up front. We have to climb a mountain and on the way, my grandmother begins to cry. She doesn't want to go up, she is in her dotage. We try to convince her. She falls.
>
> (55th session)

Associations: "My grandmother is very traditional. She is always submissive to her husband and always an excellent housewife. She is distant and not very affectionate. I remember the Japanese legend about carrying the old people to die on the mountainside. My grandmother is already very old. I believe she will not last out very long."

Interpretation: The grandmother represents the ancient outdated maternal attitude. On taking the driving into her own hands, the patient assumes control of her own process and leaves what is outdated behind. Here we have a relationship with the Mafia dream. Her grandmother was Italian and used to tell stories about the Mafia. In this way, it would seem that the patient begins to face the parental complexes by taking it on herself to drive her own life "car."

Dream:

> I am fighting with a man. He seems to be a man of wax. His belly is gaping open, and I can see his intestines and his heart. I pick up a chalice, and I drink his blood. He tells me that if I drink of his blood, I will know his name, and that if I tell everyone, he will lose his power.

> (57th session)

Associations: "It reminds me of a fairy tale where the princess has to discover the name of the dwarf so that he will not take away her child. I never saw anything resembling this dream. It seems like something very profound and strange."

Interpretation: A lack of references and the strange feeling as to this material raise the hypothesis that the dream refers to contents that are very unconscious. On entering into contact with the "blood", i.e. with the essence of this complex, its significance comes to the surface, probably associated with the paternal figure.

This interpretation was confirmed with successive analysis of diverse situations relived with the father. The patient gradually became aware of the intense relationship that she had with him and the extent to which she had shaped herself to resemble him.

In this period, the patient at times complained of pain in the region operated on and experienced fantasies of being run over or of being in the hospital and of dying.

While working with active imagination, I asked her to concentrate on the operated region and try to see what was happening. The patient soon related a scene in which her leg was being stung by many insects, causing great itching. The patient associated the mosquitoes with burns and her father's going away. Each insect had a name. It was necessary to discover each of them.

In the subsequent attempt at active imagination, the patient concentrates again on the operated region and afterward reports the following:

I was walking alone along the beach. I was very sad. I had no one to talk with. My father had gone away. I wanted him to come fetch me to play with him in the ocean, as he had always done before. But he didn't come. I walked and walked; I don't know how I stepped on the jellyfish. It startled me. I wanted my father. I wanted him to come save me. I went back home, but my mother didn't know where he was. I thought that this pain might bring him back. But it didn't work. I cried a lot. I thought that my surgery [on the melanoma] would bring him back, but that didn't work either. A birthmark looks like a burn, don't you think so? When it began to itch and burn, I now remember that I thought of my father. I also thought that if my ex- fiancé found out that I had cancer, he would pity me and return."

The memory of the fantasies that occurred when the cancer was diagnosed begins to emerge and we now realize more clearly the relationship between the burn, the paternal rejection, and the melanoma. Just as the patient had fantasized as a child that her father would return to cure her, thus as an adult, feeling rejected by her fiancé (father), the same symbol (melanoma/burn) emerges to express this suffering and the attempt to recover paternal love.

The shadow, in the guise of a needy and abandoned girl child, also becomes more conscious, as we could observe through a series of dreams containing the maternal figure and babies. In most of them, there is difficulty giving birth or the baby dies.

Dreams:

My mother gave birth and died. The baby is healthy. She knew she was going to die and for this reason she had everything ready.

My cousin was going in for an abortion.

A friend is pregnant: she tells me she feels awful.

A man attacks a woman with a knife. She runs through the house in an attempt to open the doors, but has a certain amount of difficulty with the locks. She finally emerges out in the street. When I look from the street up at a window, I can see my mother at a window up above in my grandmother's house. She covers her face with her hands. There is a great deal of suffering in her countenance.

(65th, 66th, and 67th sessions)

Associations: "My cousin has had several abortions. I would like to get pregnant. I even tried to get pregnant, to hold onto my fiancé, but he realized this and took care. I have no patience with children, and I don't believe I shall ever have children. I was annoyed when my friend got pregnant. I am not in the least sorry about her suffering. My father hurt my mother a lot."

Other dreams of similar content:

> My daughter died: I was single.
>
> I am changing her diaper for the first time. I think of leaving the window open so that she will catch a cold and die. I can see her going down and drowning.
>
> My daughter is grown up. She is run over and dies.

Associations: "My mother uses me for her own needs. She is selfish and only thinks of herself. She is not concerned about what I might need. Ever since my father left, I became company for her. Everything is to do with me. I am sorry, for her, but it annoys me. I cannot leave the house, nor have any friends. I can't stand it any longer."

Interpretation: The constellation of the maternal complex brings to the surface negative material, hate in relation to the child and towards the mother. As "her father's daughter," she rejects maternity, here associated with the shadow. Through this dream material and its associations, we can observe that in the shadow of this patient there is a destitute, rejected and abandoned little girl.

There follows a succession of dreams, fantasies and thoughts where the prime content is her own destruction.

Dreams:

> I am in a hospital. There is a girl seated crying. I go up to comfort her. The blood from her wound squirts in my face. I can taste blood.
>
> I can see I. (a friend). She has a rare disease: it seems to be progressive muscular dystrophy.
>
> I died. Somebody advises my mother. I believe it is I myself who bring her the news. First I tell her that I have suffered an accident, so that she will gradually get used to the idea of my dying.

Associations: "The sensation of being weak, ill. Devoid of energy. I. is an unhappy, lonely person."

There follows the remembrance of scenes in which she had been rejected and used by her mother. The patient feels her vitality is gone. She constantly fantasizes a recurrence of the illness. The patient continues to be depressed and lacking energy for any activity. Resigned to her failure, she constantly wishes to die. She imagines herself dying in the most diverse ways.

The positive transferential relation to the psychotherapist is the patient's only link to love, and, according to her, is what keeps her from killing herself.

In the following dream, we have a reference to this stage of the process:

> I am with D. (therapist) in a tank filled with water. The water is in movement making waves. D. compares this movement with a dream about the sea.
>
> (85th session)

We might say that this dream is in reference to the first. In this way, we would be in the center of the process, where the waves met. The fact it is a tank in place of the sea is positive, for it is indicative of a more controlled, more conscious situation, built by humans.

Dream:

> On the right side of my forehead, I have an enormous abnormal growth, which looks like a mushroom. The doctor is thinking about removing it.
>
> (87th session)

Association: "Can it be that I'll get another tumor?"

During the week of this dream, a gynecological exam turns up a cyst[4] on the right breast.

According to the doctor, the cyst's characteristics and the results of some exams indicate that it is probably malignant.

At first the patient reacted with panic and fear of death; later, with relief. The emergence of this cyst caused her emotional pain to diminish. There were moments when, to her surprise, she forgot about the emotional pain.

We raised the hypothesis that her psyche already knew of the existence of a tumor before it was visible. However, since in the dream it was a mushroom, we thought at the time that it would be less threatening; perhaps merely a temporary growth, fragile, as are mushrooms.

And, most importantly, it grew out of her head, reinforcing the hypothesis that it was of emotional origin.

Soon after, she had this dream:

> A baby (a few days old) is brought back to life when a doctor spreads cream over its body.

(89th session)

Association: "I don't want surgery or cuts, what I need is affection. The sensation of cream being spread by the doctor is one of relief and of freshness. It is as though I were burned and with the cream, I felt better."

Interpretation: This dream refers to her lack of a father. Here the doctor is the figure of the father who brings the baby back to life, rendering conscious the shadow of a little girl abandoned.

The patient began to perceive her transferential relationship to her oncologist. She wanted the doctor to pay attention to her as a daughter, and simultaneously she felt that he wanted to "cut" her, immediately recommending surgery and advising her, were the tumor to prove to be cancerous, to remove her ovaries as a preventive measure. She felt the doctor was like her father, objective and removed, quickly doing what was needed without concern for feelings.

The patient reacted to her doctor's orientation with despair. She was young, still dreamed of marrying and having children. These surgeries (breast and ovaries) would certainly mutilate her. She consulted her father about the situation, and he took an attitude similar to that of the doctor.

Dreams:

> A man is driving along arm in arm with a woman. Somebody shoots and kills the woman. The bullet travels through the windshield.
>
> I have eggs of various animals that are beginning to hatch. I have two small caimans and an assortment of snakes, of which I am afraid. I don't exactly know what to do about them. I put the caimans into a lake near my house, with a net over them so they won't attack anyone.
>
> My arms and chest are all covered with green crabs. I scream in horror for someone to help me, but nobody comes.

(93rd session)

Associations: "Fear of the biopsy and of the surgery. I cannot keep up a relationship. I am always killed in the end. A man will always wound me. Children today are caimans. They come from eggs, not from the womb. Caimans and snakes are reminiscent of primitive animals that kill in cold blood. They are in a lake close to the house. That's where I am going to die, never having given birth to anything. I have bred only snakes and lizards. I don't trust my doctor."

Interpretation: Mutilation would be viewed by the patient as the death of maternity, of the possibility of getting married and of having children. Here the patient realizes how vital these desires are and how mutilation of the body is associated with her shadow.

The needy and abandoned girl child had to die because it was not cared for. She now realizes that if she wishes to live she will have to change her attitude immediately and take care of her "child" without passing the child to others to care for.

Also, Cecilia re-experiences through the doctor the wound of paternal abandonment by feeling the doctor to be an aggressive and destructive man and, at the same time, that she pushes him into this role. The offspring are destructive reptiles that may well turn against her who first produced them. There is no maternal identification, nor the present possibility of breastfeeding since the offspring are not mammals. All takes place at an extremely primitive and archetypal level. On the other hand, the fact the eggs hatched is a possibility of contact with the contents that were formerly unconscious.

Parallel to this, owing to the negative transferential relationship established with the doctor, the patient was forwarded to a gynecologist. She was more understanding and requested a new batch of tests.

In therapy the emergence of maternal contents becomes pronounced. The patient feels that her body is against her. She feels that she will die because her body doesn't like her. I ask her to use active imagination to try to talk with her body and ask why it wants to destroy her.

The image of a gigantic woman appeared. This woman was terrible and hated her. The patient tried to escape. Wherever she ran, the earth opened up into craters. As she tried to hide behind some boulders, rain and lightening bolts fell on her. She left therapy deeply afraid and without any resolution. No dialogue was possible (107th session).

The patient then drew the witch-woman (Figure 5.3) and saw that she was powerless against this terrible woman who desired the

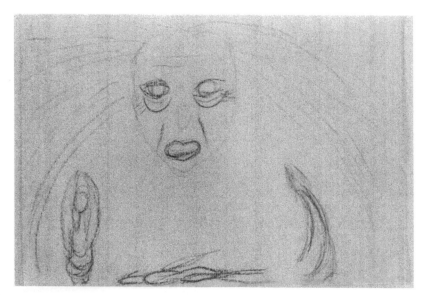

Figure 5.3 Patient's "witch-woman" drawing. (A full-color version of this figure can be viewed at http://www.brunner-routledge.co.uk/ramos)

patient's death simply because the witch was evil. There was no escape. The patient would die in any event. The maternal complex, in its negative aspect, elicited the maternal archetype, also in its negative aspect as the witch–mother figure. The destructive mother, present in the body of her daughter, wanted the daughter's destruction. The three women who appear in the drawing are the patient trying to talk with the giant and then, finding her effort in vain, the patient giving up and preparing to die. How could she fight against the witch–mother invading the daughter's own body? It was as if the cells of her body had revolted against her. How can you identify the enemy when it is part of yourself, when it is your mother? Some cells tried to destroy the patient; how could she identify them?

In Figure 5.4, the patient has sketched herself lying down, defeated, with an enormous bleeding wound threatening to crush her. At first glimpse, she imagined it to be an open breast, with dark spots inside. But then she saw that the spots looked like birds gathering, ready to fly. She reinforced the forms with black ink and took heart at the newly emerged symbol. Even without understanding it, she felt it to be positive.

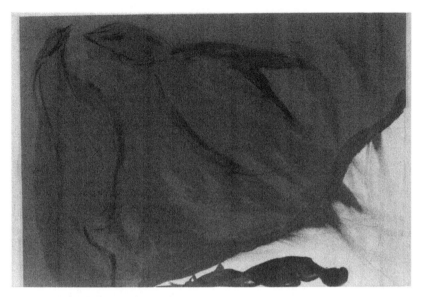

Figure 5.4 Patient's drawing of two birds and a woman. (A full-color version of this figure can be viewed at http://www.brunner-routledge.co.uk/ramos)

In this period, owing to her intense anguish in face of the biopsy that was to be completed, the patient had daily sessions for five days.

Figure 5.5, drawn in one of the following sessions, results from the suggestion of imagining the cyst in her right breast. The drawing represents the same crushed and defeated woman, imprisoned among the lactiferous ducts. "Nothing can flow from my breasts. They are clogged up. There's no milk, just blood. I have no energy to rise. The woman is crushed. I need help."

But who could help her?

Dreams at this stage reveal intense suffering:

> A family is seated around a table. A man comes up with a small net, and in it a species of red insect. He says the insect, just by being near, would kill all around it. First they would feel dry in the mouth, and they would burn to death. The father attempts to run away to plead for help; however, the man runs after him and catches him. Only the maid manages to escape.
>
> I suffered a car accident. I broke my right arm, but I am bandaged from the waist up. I ask them to call my ex-fiancé, but they cannot get through.

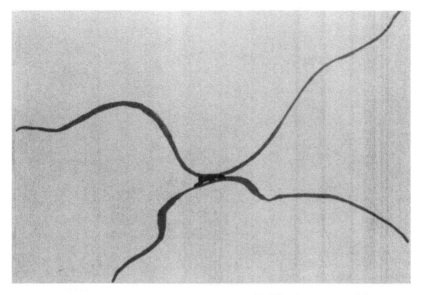

Figure 5.5 Patient's drawing of a "defeated" woman. (A full-color version of this figure can be viewed at http://www.brunner-routledge.co.uk/ramos)

> My family and myself have our wrists cut; however, there is no blood. My cut is the deepest.
>
> (109th session)

Associations: A feeling of being broken, wounded. The maid is the simplest person, but the most direct. She says what she thinks and cries for any reason.

Interpretation: It is not possible to take up the link with the fiancé once more, nor with her parents, who have aged and are weak. The maid is her most expressive and direct shadow aspect, which must be rendered aware, for only she can save. The insect reminds us of the first dream with insects and a burn. Are we in the middle of the process?

Figure 5.6 is a reply to the question "who could help?" There appears here a "devouring monster." "He will eat the tumor. Only he can combat the witch. Only another equal to her could defeat her." The crushed woman continues in the lower right corner of the drawing, now praying and asking for help. According to the patient, the monster is not benevolent; it merely wants to thwart the witch, and therefore will help her. "He eats the tumor."

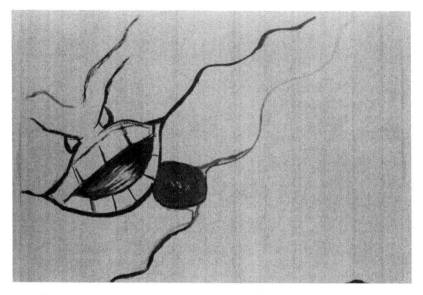

Figure 5.6 Patient's drawing of a monster and a tumor. (A full-color version of this figure can be viewed at http://www.brunner-routledge.co.uk/ramos)

I ask the patient to imagine, several times per day, the monster devouring her cyst. The patient repeats the image frequently (five to six times per day) and says she feels heat in the cyst's region.

Within the breast of Figure 5.7 we have an oval personage between the ducts, in the region of the cyst. The body is that of the monster, but the head is a caricature. "I like him. He's funny. He has a sense of humor and controls the monster. The monster ate the tumor already, it's just that he could feel himself powerful and got out of control, attacked me as did the witch. But here he can do nothing, because the guy on top is laughing and putting him in the proper perspective. He says the monster gives no orders. It is transformed into Tipsy Fool [an inflatable weighted toy], who gets pushed from one side to the other, but doesn't give any orders."

Cecilia started to realize that her emotional reaction to the loss of her boyfriend was tragic out of all proportion to what had really happened. That reaction had been much more an acting-out of the pain of parental abandonment, and thus she might develop a certain sense of humor and laugh when remembering certain "tragic" scenes with her ex-fiancé. She was able to see herself as a person who had

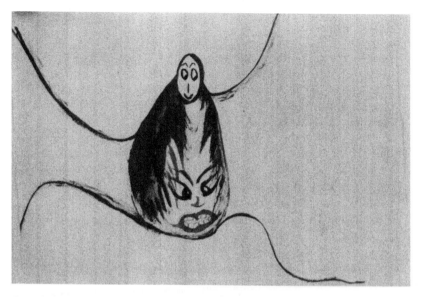

Figure 5.7 Patient's drawing of a "funny personage." (A full-color version of this figure can be viewed at http://www.brunner-routledge.co.uk/ramos)

now discovered her role and why she had been compulsively drawn to repeat certain patterns. It emerged ever more clearly that the unconsciousness of suffering, due as much to the maternal as to the paternal complex, both of them negative, had made the suffering impossible to express on a conscious, verbal plane and therefore caused its expression on a more concrete and corporal plane.

The mammary cyst was the cyst of the maternal relationship, which had "clogged up" her relation with the feminine/maternal and, at the same time, was an expression of that dysfunction.

The leg cyst was the cyst of the paternal relationship, its corporal identification with the rejecting father.

Dream:

> A child falls into the water. She was playing on the ice when it broke. I run to help, and stretch out on the ice so that it will not break and give my hand to the child. I ask someone to hold on to my feet so as to make a chain.

> (110th session)

Association: "I was on the ice. Now I feel as if I were emerging, but it is not at all easy. I am afraid to dive and not to make it up to the surface again."

Interpretation: We can see here the child on the ice with her shadow aspect wounded, without affection, which still runs the risk of being killed. Her desire, however, is to save the child.

When she has to fight for her life, the patient assumes an active attitude and makes an effort to survive. We remember the "cold" here that she felt at her father's leaving home.

Two days after this image and this dream, the biopsy revealed that the cyst was benign. The doctor attributed the different diagnosis to an error of the previous doctor. The patient attributed it to the analytic work carried out. The question remains open as to whether or not the intense analytic work of this period brought about an alteration on the cellular level.

Dream:

> I am at sea. The waves are strong, but I manage to swim. I have to contend with the waves a great deal so as not to drown. Someone throws a tennis ball at me hard. The ball strikes me on the breast, and I break a rib. We are on a distant beach. I find a telephone on the road, but do not know the name of the beach so as to advise the police. Finally someone tells me the name of the beach. I get home. My wound is sore. My mother is sad. I ask her what the matter is? She says that my father is very ill, in hospital. I did not worry, for I remembered that a clairvoyant had told me it would be an attack of no importance. I thought of visiting him to make use of the occasion and to care for myself.
>
> (120th session)

Associations: "A tennis ball – I learned how to play tennis with my father. It's a sport he likes. I have suffered ever since I was a child with fantasies of this type where my father or else my mother was sick or dead."

Interpretation: This dream makes clear reference to the first dream where, following great effort and several wounds, the patient manages to leave for a new beach. Reflecting on the present situation, we might say the patient is through the most conflicting stage of the process. She has yet to deal with the wound produced by aggressivity and paternal rejection (the tennis ball). The place where the father is (in hospital) is the most appropriate for this purpose, without there being apparently greater risk.

In subsequent sessions, the paternal figure is worked out in depth. Dream:

> I am in a car driven by a man, my boyfriend. We try to get the car out of the snow, but it skids with wheels held fast. It goes forwards and backwards. Only with great effort do we set the car free and get out of the snow.
>
> (131st session)

Association: "I do not know the boy in the car. He seems to me to be strong and good-looking."

Interpretation: Here there arises the figure of the positive animus who drives and warms, for it is through his ability that the patient comes in from the "cold" and the possibility of a new life emerges. Probably, the liberation of the negative paternal complex rendered possible a connection through to the animus, as also to the conscious awareness of the rejected child formerly situated in the shadow. This reminds us of the dream about the child who falls into a frozen lake, and the figure of the Indian (animus) killed by the police (father).

The patient described how at this stage, for the first time, she engaged in an intellectual fight with a colleague and, to her surprise, upheld ideas different from those she had up to then.

The image of the child who needs to be cared for and supported was worked on intensively. The patient realized that when she didn't take care of "her," the pain in the region of the scar appeared, as well as fantasies of cancer and death.

In the concluding sessions of this process, the patient was better able to elaborate the relation between the unconscious and the insufficient expression of her conflicts, and how these factors led to the formation of her organic symptoms.

The information available to me, two years after her discharge, is that the patient is well, working, participating actively in a social group, and does not present any further symptoms.

There were a total of 167 sessions spread over two and a half years, with an average of two sessions per week.

We can look at this case, like the previous ones, at various levels.

At the most superficial level, as a personality trait, this patient fits into Type C: an apparently well-intentioned person, helpful, always ready to sacrifice herself for others. Present in this patient are difficulty in expressing anger and an attitude of resigned defeat, which are identified by others' research as frequent in patients with melanoma and other types of cancer.

On the other hand, the patient, after the break-up of her romance, underwent an experience we may categorize as chronic stress, because, as we have seen, this event was a re-experience of her father's abandoning her. The fact that she could not, at the time, express her sentiments turned her suffering unconscious and chronic.

At the most profound level, we verify the existence of two negative complexes taking part in the formation of her organic symptoms, namely the negative maternal and paternal complexes. Both expressed themselves symbolically at the bodily pole as symptoms, given that unconscious mechanisms impeded their integration into consciousness. The following schemes help us to summarize partially the great number of images produced by this patient (Figures 5.8, 5.9 and 5.10).

Central symbols of the process

If we take the disease "melanoma" as a symbol, we can clearly see its significance in this process. Wrapped up in painful mourning, the patient relives abandonment by her father through the abandonment by her fiancé, and reopens a wound coincident with her paternal identification. The "spots" take on the sense of a link to her father, and we might interpret their malignancy as the malignancy of the paternal relationship.

Curiously, the need for an operation indicates the need to wipe out this identification. Since this wiping out cannot take place on an

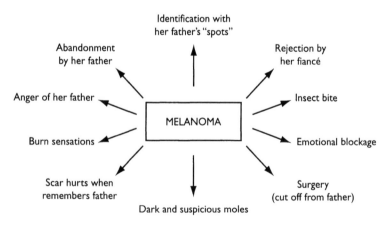

Figure 5.8 Case summary of "the depressive" (with respect to melanoma).

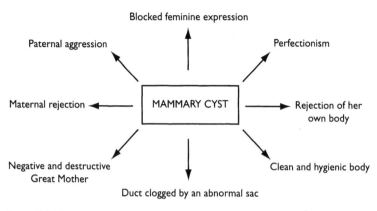

Figure 5.9 Case summary of "the depressive" (with respect to mammary cyst).

abstract level, it happens concretely in the body. The fantasies and dreams of the patient at the time of the surgery are proof of the paternal relation, as is also the constant pain in the scarred region when remembering her father painfully.

It is interesting for us to observe here the partial congruence of the symbol "melanoma" with the paternal complex (Figures 5.8 and 5.10), as well as the congruence of the symbol "mammary cyst" with the maternal complex (Figures 5.9 and 5.10). The various common features confirm that both symbols are expressions of the negative paternal complexes.

The shadow (Figure 5.10) expresses itself in the symbols of the injured, sick, and dead girls, unconscious to the patient, who in her persona appeared independent and always ready to help (never needed anything, never had any problem). Here the shadow is active within the body as organic symptoms, showing how serious the injury has been.

Regarding the mammary cyst (Figure 5.9), we were able to see how the negative maternal complex activated the archetype of the Great Mother in its negative aspect, threatening the body's existence. As it affected an essentially maternal area, the patient was forced to affirm a desire that had been denied until then: the desire to be a mother. While previously she had belittled and ridiculed this desire, partially because of identification with the father, now she was forced to struggle for its fulfillment, if she wished to experience this archetype as a mother.

The struggle against the negative Great Mother took place on various levels, but the turning point came with the aid of the

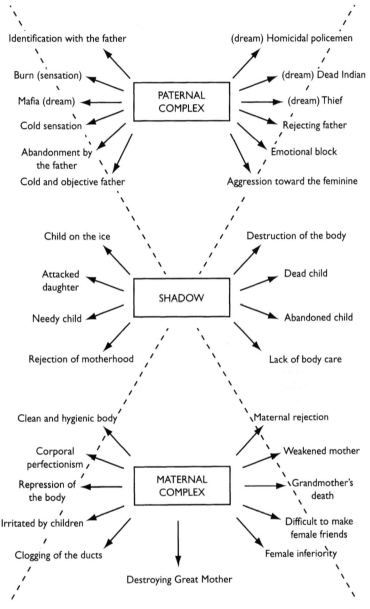

Figure 5.10 Overall case summary of "the depressive," incorporating mother complex, shadow and father complex.

archetype of the Father. The emergence of a masculine archetypal symbol, the figure of the "devouring monster," signifies a struggle between the parental archetypes, necessary if the patient was not to stay totally under the thrall of the evil mother.

The process seems to come under conscious control when the patient realizes that she can also control the unconscious "monster." Consequently, there emerge the figures of the positive animus and logos.

At this point the patient takes ownership of the process, without, however, considering that her power is relative. Later, she realizes that keeping her psychological balance will depend on constant renewal of the link between ego and Self, through the emerging images. She also realizes that this is the best, and perhaps only, prophylactic against unconscious invasions on the most varied levels.

Repressed anger becomes a revolt listened to, but not communicated. Wherever it is present, it is active, creating destructive behavior out of control. Since there is no vent for externalizing it, repressed anger will act in some form, synchronistically at the unconscious organic and psychic levels.

The deeper structures, at the infrared pole of the instinctual spectrum, are where we will find repressed anger, turning against that which keeps it prisoner in the body. Friend and enemy get mixed up. Once again we observe the disease as having an evolutionary goal, forcing the individual to contact the unknown and expand her consciousness.

Chapter 6

The symbolic body

Case vignettes

> The body knows things a long time before the mind catches up with them. I was wondering what my body knew that I didn't.
>
> (Kidd, 2002: 69)

Various cases have been treated using the analytic model. We will present here, as examples, principal moments in the process of six patients with different symptoms. As mentioned above, one of the main aims is to develop techniques that allow for brief therapy, focused on the illness, to be used with hospitalized patients or those who wish to get rid of the disease and are not interested in deeper analysis. Nevertheless, healing presumes an awareness of certain conflicts and of unconscious mechanisms, so that brief therapy is not always possible. The time of treatment depends largely on the ego conditions of the patient facing the power of complexes and defense mechanisms that surround the symptom.

The repressed person: when the skin erupts (acne rosacea)[1]

Daniel, a 36-year-old public relations man, had been afflicted with allergic symptoms and other dermatological problems ever since he was a child. At around 22 years of age he received the diagnosis of acne rosacea, a chronic skin disorder that affected most of his face and was characterized by redness and inflammation.

His job was adversely affected, as it depended very much on physical appearance to please the clients, and for days he had been ashamed of showing himself in public. He underwent various skin treatments that resulted in temporary relief. Daniel was aware that the symptoms worsened after family fights. Usually quiet and introverted, Daniel did not react to brotherly provocations and always tried to keep fights among his brothers from getting out of hand. Quite a few times, he intervened to keep them from getting more aggressive towards each other. He was considered a family mediator and was called on many times to intervene in conflict situations. According to Daniel, his marriage was fine; his wife was very demanding but he knew how to avoid quarrels, so they could have a "harmonious marriage."

This was one of the cases that was treated in a few sessions using the sandplay technique.[2] We will relate two scenes that portray Daniel's process.

In the first scene, Daniel puts his hands on the sand, leaving deep imprints (Figure 6.1). He has the sensation that a protective uterus is there, and feels sheltered. The hand prints here also depict Daniel's recognizing his own self and taking possession of a territory. Being the middle son in a family of various siblings, he never had his own space and always gave up his place to stronger, more aggressive brothers. Daniel is moved by the image of the

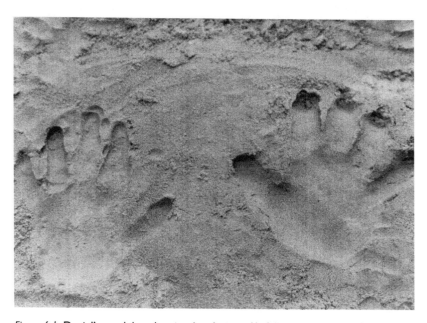

Figure 6.1 Daniel's sandplay, showing handprints. (A full-color version of this figure can be viewed at http://www.brunner-routledge.co.uk/ramos)

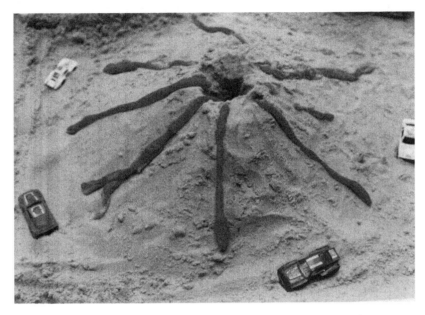

Figure 6.2 Daniel's sandplay, showing volcano. (A full-color version of this figure can be viewed at http://www.brunner-routledge.co.uk/ramos)

hands, and realizes how little they have been used to express his emotions.

In the second scene, Daniel draws a volcano spouting powerfully (Figure 6.2), and cries a lot after finishing. Around the volcano there is a racetrack. The cars race around the volcano without paying attention to the danger. The symbol of the volcano becomes central to the process, and could be seen as a metaphor for his acne.

Through it we are able to perceive how much Daniel has been repressing his emotions by always being submissive. He has had great difficulty in expressing his feelings and repressed anger, for this is how he has been raised. As a fervent Roman Catholic, he thought he should always imitate Christ by "turning the other cheek."

The cars run close to imminent danger, representing his idealized persona, which, indifferent to danger, sought always to appear calm and in control of the situation. To maintain his efficiency at work, Daniel was always smiling and showing himself to have a phlegmatic nature, which won him praise. However, Daniel now realized the acne rosacea to be an exploding volcano and the pus that ran down his face a lava of emotions he had repressed for so many years.

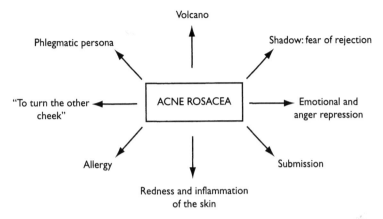

Figure 6.3 Case summary of "the repressed person" (acne rosacea).

If we understand acne rosacea as a symbol, we have the above (Figure 6.3).

Central symbol of the process

After perceiving the volcano as a liberating force for feelings repressed throughout the years, Daniel began to voice his anger, no longer serving as a mediator of family conflicts. Quite the contrary, in giving his opinions and talking of his feelings he destabilized family relations, which counted on his apparent good sense. As he began letting go of his aggression, at times actually in "volcanic crises," his skin began showing significant improvement, with his doctor putting an end to treatment. The repressed volcano had gone into erruption on his face as the best means of emotional expression found by the Self.

The conscious transduction of the physical symptom to an expression of anger, first in the sand and then verbally, allowed for a quick tuning in to his feelings and permanent relief from his symptoms.

The constipated person: when nothing is expelled (fecaloma)[3]

Elise is 54 years old, obese and apparently childish. She was sent by the doctor treating her for pneumonia, after having been examined by several other doctors due to different symptoms. Elise used to see a minimum of two doctors a week, always with varied symptoms. Her latest doctor, perceiving a lack of affection as the root of the search for attention, recommended psychotherapy. Elise did not complain of any emotional problems, stating that she suffered only from chronic constipation and shortness of breath. She only went to therapy because her doctor, whom she saw as a father figure, insisted on it. All other doctors she termed incompetent, for they "never found anything wrong."

Elise used to have fecalomas and occasionally had to go to the emergency unit to have them removed. The cause of the fecaloma was a prolonged constipation that provoked an urgent need to defecate that was impossible to carry through, causing pains in the rectum, anus and abdomen.

She was very repressed in her speech and gestures. She was afraid of letting go of her emotions and losing her affective connections. Because of this, she never fought back and let herself be abused by other people, so as not to lose them.

Elise spent the sessions describing her difficulties in going to the bathroom and conflicts with her maid. She lived alone and, apart from her domestic staff, doctors were her only other contact with other people. The maid had a central role in her life. Besides preparing her meals, she gave her injections and enemas. These became Elise's only means of physical contact in a very lonely world. Her voracious eating made her obese, a state that was aggravated by her refusal to move around. She always wanted to be served, and kept various house servants at her beck and call.

In this context, we can see her chronic constipation as physical and emotional immobility, a desire to keep everything that she could get (felt always as "too little"). On the other hand, her need to be cared for due to her health problem required that other people move her passive body and meet her unconscious desire for physical contact. Elise was a big baby, as fragile as she was heavy, insatiable and constantly calling for attention.

She didn't remember her dreams and refused to do any expressive work in therapy, showing a strong resistance in dealing with her emotional hardships. She put all the blame on the body and refused analytical interpretation. Her passive behavior was at the same time highly aggressive, with imminent risk of putting a stop to treatment. Nevertheless, Elise received with enthusiasm the idea of looking at pictures and thus we spent a few sessions going over photograph albums, recalling a totally forgotten past.

For the first time in her life Elise started talking about her parents and, in recalling her mother's rejection of her, urinated on the chair, losing control over her body. She now remembered that her mother left her in the care of various nannies, and could not recall a single instant of being caressed by her or her father. He was a highly successful doctor who traveled a lot, giving speeches throughout the world. Abandoned, Elise entertained herself with servants and could not make friends. The death of her parents worsened the situation, isolating her even more from social life.

Along with the rising recollections and the discomfort brought on by conflictive situations, Elise began to feel intestinal movements. At a certain point she said that I, her therapist, was the "best purgative, better than any medication." Many times during or after analysis she had to run out to defecate.

Central symbol of the process

Elise would traditionally be classified as an alexithymic patient, and therefore not one to undergo any psychotherapeutic treatment. However, as we saw, her body was the symbolic expression of her unconscious process: an enormous, authoritarian appearance hiding in its shadow the hurt child, abandoned and highly deprived (Figure 6.4).

Her fecaloma could be viewed as a symbolic expression of her desire to retain all she had acquired (always insufficient) and at the

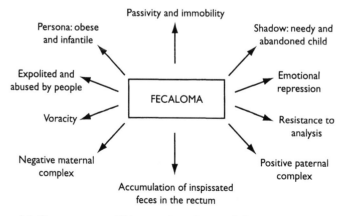

Figure 6.4 Case summary of "the constipated person" (fecaloma).

same time a paralysis, which as a secondary gain allowed her bodily contact and physical care.

Nevertheless, the awareness of these factors and the gradual strengthening of her ego, along with improvement of the intestinal system, were felt as a threat by the maid, who began to refuse to bring the patient for treatment. Despite several interviews with the maid, she was set on boycotting analysis and the patient gave up treatment through fear of losing her only companion. I found out from her doctor that around two years later, though cured of fecaloma, the patient died from respiratory problems.

The freezing hands: when we swim under ice (Reynaud's syndrome)[4]

Fiona is 32 years old and complains of cold hands and feet even during summer. During winter (average temperature 15°C where she lives) her toes are almost frozen. She cannot stand the cold. Fiona also complains of terrible back pain. She feels depressed and has not been able to succeed professionally. She remembers that ever since she was young she always needed to wear a sweater. She had difficulties sleeping because "the bed was cold." She was given the diagnosis of Reynaud's syndrome, and had already undergone various treatments with temporary results.

Fiona is very unhappy in her marriage, but remains married from fear of being alone. Her husband is an alcoholic and has mistresses, but Fiona feels weak and unable to make a decision to change her life.

Her appearance, however, is strong, muscular and highly masculine. She cannot recall ever wearing a skirt or dress in her life. She had little contact with her mother, who abandoned the family when the patient was seven years old.

In this case we have two main symbols: constant pain in the back and Reynaud's syndrome.

As the patient had already undergone various psychotherapeutic treatments and was familiar with active imagination, after a few preliminary sessions we used this technique, aiming to reach her symptoms directly.

Back pain

With her eyes closed, Fiona reported the following image:

> I am riding a very tall horse. I don't want to get on the horse but my father is making me do so. I am very afraid. The horse bolts and I hold onto his neck. I feel very frightened.

The patient had completely forgotten this situation. Remembering it, she became very angry with her father and at the same time she felt an acute pain in her back and neck. We perceived here the activation of a complex that synchronously produces an image and a pain.

The father always demanded that she be a hero. As the eldest of three children she always had to be the first in all activities. She was a model student and sports player. She worked hard at getting first place, which happened frequently.

We could say that her father complex was in the contracted muscle in her back that protected her from a "deadly fall."

Reynaud's syndrome

Image:

> I am swimming in a frozen lake under the ice. I try to come up but I can't find the way out. I feel more and more frozen.

During this exercise the patient became increasingly pale. Her fingers turned light blue. As much as I (the analyst) tried to break the ice, nothing seemed to help. We thought of a pick to break the ice but the patient did not have the strength to hold it. I also felt cold. There was as well the risk of the pick hurting her, for it was not possible to know for sure what her position was in the water, under the ice. In her imagination the patient was suffering and felt that she could die as she saw no way out of this dangerous situation.

On the other side, on top of the ice, I also felt impotent, not knowing how to help her. Then it occurred to me to move close to the patient's hand (without touching) to try to warm her. Of course! It was the heat (love) and not the pick that could melt the ice. The pick would have been a very aggressive solution (more masculine and logical). I realized that I also had to break the ice and move closer. I could only help her if I was able to transmit my warmth rather than interpretations that only reaffirmed her sense of abandonment and strengthened her positive father complex (positive here in the sense that she was extremely linked and dedicated to her father, trying to imitate him in all possible ways). The feminine, maternal side had been repressed together with ambiguous feelings regarding the abandoning mother.

Central symbol of the process

In this case we can see clearly that the two organic symptoms were linked with the father and mother complexes (Figure 6.5). In the shadow, compensating for the efficient, professional and winning sportswoman, remained the girl almost frozen from lack of affection and warmth. While the back pain expressed the authoritarian, demanding father complex, Reynaud's syndrome mirrored the coldness of her affective relations, of which the patient was not conscious. In the transduction of this symptom to the ice image, the

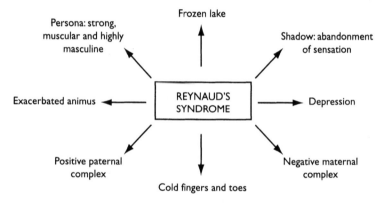

Figure 6.5 Case summary of "the freezing hands" (Reynaud's syndrome).

patient was able to express the grief that she denied in her mother's abandonment. Exercises following this image, where the patient saw herself giving love and warmth to the child of her imagination (shadow), slowly alleviated her symptoms until they were gone.

The untouchable princess: when sexual instinct threatens (pelvic inflammatory disease)[5]

Georgia, 42 years old, suffered from recurrent gynecological infections without her doctors being able to discover the cause or how the patient was always getting infected. The gynecologist's main hypothesis was that the patient suffered from some immunological weakening that left her prone to these infections. However, it was intriguing that this disturbance only manifested itself in the genital system. She was referred to me by her doctor, who thought she was depressed.

Georgia seems a princess, floating and untouched. She looks very young but is expressionless. Her beautiful hands call attention; it is as if they were never used. The patient actually comes from a very rich family and has never done any domestic activities. She spends her day reading novels and dreaming that a strong man will one day come and rescue her from her dull life.

In the beginning she did not complain of any conflict. Her only problem was her terrible fear of dogs. She avoided walking on the streets for fear of them.

Georgia was also very religious. Every day she went to a spiritual center and to church for the communion service. Her marriage was "normal," in her own words, and she said she had sexual relations with her husband only to please him, for she felt no pleasure in the activity.

This case was treated with the sandplay technique. In the beginning, Georgia avoided touching the sand so as not to "dirty my hands." With time, she became less inhibited and moved the sand freely. Concurrently, she began to learn to cook, showing great pleasure especially in working with meat. She brought me a turnover made with her own hands, with great pride.

Two main scenes illustrate this process, as follows.

> A dog is talking to a girl and a strong, fat Buddha (Figure 6.6). The dog asks the Buddha to get out of the doorway of the house so that the girl can come and play with him in the forest. The Buddha says that the girl cannot come out; she has to stay inside praying and meditating.
>
> A prostitute, a woman in red, is upset because the priest will not let her enter the church (Figure 6.7). There is an abandoned baby under a fruit tree. The baby is crying from hunger, but he can't eat the fruit. There are some big insects behind the rock that might attack the baby.

We can see in these two scenes that the patient's father complex (represented by the priest and the Buddha) prevents her from leaving, from going to the forest to play. Here the dog represents her instinctive and sexual life that threatens her, and the girl is her

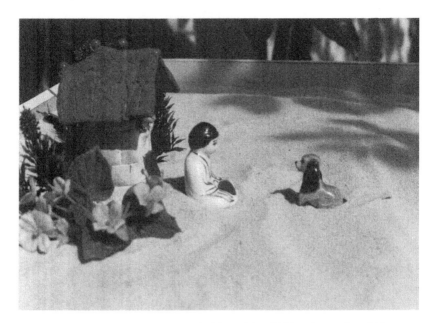

Figure 6.6 Georgia's sandplay, showing Buddha and dog. (A full-color version of this figure can be viewed at http://www.brunner-routledge.co.uk/ramos)

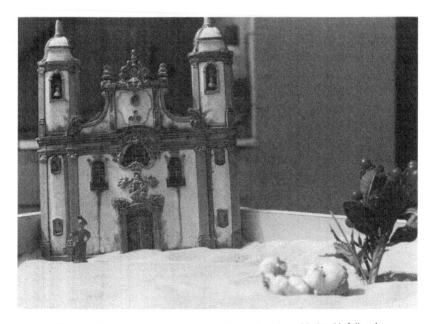

Figure 6.7 Georgia's sandplay, showing prostitute, church and baby. (A full-color version of this figure can be viewed at http://www.brunner-routledge.co.uk/ramos)

shadow imprisoned by religious authority. Her shadow also appears as a prostitute and abandoned baby. She feared that liberating her sexuality would transform her into a prostitute.

When we worked with the dog symbolism her fantasy was that it would jump panting on her breast, without biting her. Through active imagination we realized that this image caused a certain sexual excitement that left her quite disoriented. She actually remembered a small dog in her childhood that used to masturbate itself on the furniture and once ejaculated on her leg. Slowly, the patient was able, to her surprise, to perceive the sensuality of her own body and other sensations of which she had never been aware.

Central symbol of the process

The transduction of the organic polarity symptoms was helped here by work in the sand, where the patient could concretely deal with her unconscious conflicts (Figure 6.8).

Various dreams followed these representations. Georgia was able to see that her extreme religiosity was a defense mechanism against sensuality and eroticism. Coming from a highly traditional, strict family, she had had a convenience marriage and now was ready to reevaluate her life. She took up gardening on realizing the great pleasure she got from messing with earth. There were no more

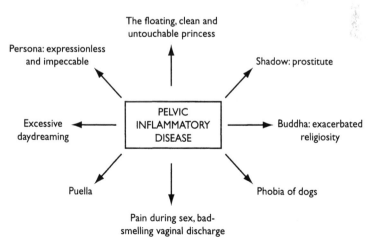

Figure 6.8 Case summary of "the untouchable princess" (pelvic inflammatory disease).

infections, according to her doctor, two years following the end of therapy.

The guilty person: when the head is tortured (migraine)[6]

Helen, a 49-year-old woman, was a famous professor who had suffered from migraine headaches for about ten years, treated with various procedures giving only temporary relief. Although she was taking the most modern drugs for this illness, at least three times a month she was unable to work or even to open her eyes.

Evolution of the analysis

The patient had a deep maternal wound. At the age of 14 she had discovered that she was the daughter of her mother's lover. However, she recollected that even as a very small child she had noticed her mother's affairs. She was always terrified that her "lawful" father would discover them and murder her mother, because he had a violent personality. Her mother had forced her to be her silent accomplice, a fact that was hard for her to reveal even in analysis.

She refused to get married but had many affairs, always breaking up the relationship upon falling in love with another man. Usually she got interested in married men until she succeeded in getting them to wreck their marriages.

During the analysis we were able to work with her hatred of men and of her mother. She had a strong, seductive defense mechanism and, at the same time, identified strongly with her mother.

During an acute migraine incident, I asked her to close her eyes and increase the pain in her head.

Helen grew redder and redder, and the veins on her forehead became very prominent. Suddenly she opened her startled eyes, saying:

> I was in a village, being judged in a public square. Someone squeezed my head with a tourniquet to make me confess my guilt.

Helen returns to the torture scene and screams to all that she is not guilty. But she rids herself of the tourniquet only when she denounces the truly guilty party: her mother. As she does so, to my surprise, the color of her skin returns to normal and the patient attains complete and immediate relief from her migraine.

Of course, the migraine returns in a few days. But, after she confesses other "guilt" feelings, her symptoms gradually fade until they disappear completely.

Central symbol of the process

This was an extremely serious situation and therapy ran for three years (Figure 6.9). The repressed suffering and terrible fear of what discovery of the betrayal might entail created in the patient a constant feeling that a bomb might explode at any second. Helen remembered that on coming home at night she was so afraid that her father might discover the truth that she would hide in bed with terrible headaches. She also feared that her looking like her biological father would betray the situation and thus tried to change her looks to the maximum, hiding her face with hair and big glasses. At the same time she hated men, whom she blamed for the confusion and anguish in her life. She used her seductive powers (gained from her mother) to get money and destroy her companions, acting out a type of "Don Juanism" of which she was initially very proud.

The migraine here was the symbol that best expressed all her complexes. Helen later told that she had to control her memories and lies so as not to confuse herself, and that many times she could not remember what she had said. This lying behavior, used in the beginning consciously, became with time a defense mechanism, which

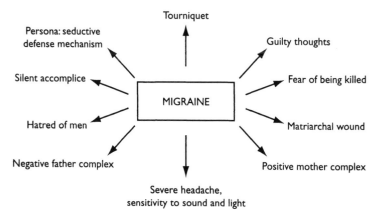

Figure 6.9 Case summary of "the guilty person" (migraine).

protected the patient from a possible death situation. For, within her perception, due to her complicity she would be killed along with her mother. While involuntary, this complicity, even though it protected her mother, generated an unconscious feeling of guilt that tortured the patient. Her organic symptom could only be relieved when she denounced the original conflict and told of the traumatic situation in which she lived. Permanent relief took more sessions due to intense feelings of terror and hatred associated with this. The defense mechanisms surrounding the symptom protected the patient from a deeper pain: that of being herself betrayed by her mother, who used and abused her love and loyalty.

The dirty uterus: when incest is remembered (miscarriage)[7]

Isabel was 28 years old and had had successive miscarriages. In the past six years she had suffered four spontaneous abortions. During the past two pregnancies she had been bedridden, under the care of medical specialists. Nevertheless, in the sixth month of pregnancy she lost the babies. Clinical exams on the fetus and on the mother were unable to detect any organic problems that could explain what had occurred.

We worked with imagination and, with her eyes closed, Isabel, in touch with her body, "saw" a smelly, dirty uterus. During an exercise of imagination she visualized that she pulled a rope from within her uterus. Slowly coming out with the rope were pieces of a noxious and putrid fetus.

At this moment Isabel started to remember that when she was a child her mother put her to sleep after lunch in the same room with her grandfather. She recalled that her grandfather fondled her and obliged her to fondle him also (she had forgotten these facts completely).

At first she thought the situation pleasurable but as time passed, the grandfather became more abusive and she did not want to lie down with him anymore. As the mother did not understand her behavior, she had to obey and go to "sleep." Isabel remembered subsequently that when she was not able to sleep her maid used to masturbate her to calm her down (at about six to seven years of age).

Today all these situations are remembered with repugnance and revulsion. Another fact is also significant: When Isabel was 12 she saw her father kissing the maid. The father denied the fact and the mother accused her of trying to destroy her marriage. Nevertheless, the father later left the house to marry the then pregnant maid.

All these facts were extremely painful to the patient. Many times she thought that she had hallucinated and that she was going crazy. Other times she thought that she was bad and mean. How could she have such bad thoughts about such nice people? She felt that the dirt was in herself, not in other people. Isabel felt also that her uterus was the place that was bad and dirty because it was there that the "crime" had happened. Nothing good could live there. Her uterus was contaminated and rotten.

Central symbol of the process

The therapy consisted of "cleaning the uterus" through imagination techniques and relieving the repressed unconscious emotions associated with the images that started to pour out. Memories of incest and lies, which hid illicit sexual situations, were the filth that contaminated her uterus.

After eight months of therapy Isabel got pregnant and had a normal pregnancy. She refused to rest and take hormones. She felt now that her uterus was a clean and beautiful nest where a baby could grow and live. Today she has three healthy children.

We see in this case the power of the symbolic body in the form of the pregnant and contaminated uterus. This image impregnated in the patient's organism informed her that there was no place for pregnancy, for her uterus was already filled by a decomposing fetus. The

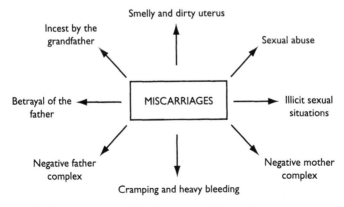

Figure 6.10 Case summary of "the dirty uterus" (miscarriage).

gross feeling and the rejection of all that was linked to the uterus were mirrored in various involuntary abortions. No matter how much she wished for a child, the memory registered in her body's cells defensively avoided a new traumatic situation. We could even say that the abortions were a defense protecting Isabel from an "incestuous pregnancy," in that her being was highly contaminated by incestuous and abusive relations.

Chapter 7

Conclusions

> Our little Spaceship Earth is only eight thousand miles in diameter,
> which is almost a negligible dimension in the great vastness of
> space . . . Spaceship Earth was so extraordinarily well invented and
> designed that to our knowledge humans have been on board it for
> two million years not even knowing that they were on board a ship
> . . . Now there is one outstandingly important fact regarding
> Spaceship Earth, and that is that no instruction book came with it.
>
> (Fuller, 1963: 4)

We were able to observe, in the cases described in Chapters 5 and 6,
that when an emotion was evoked or expressed, a physiological
change also took place. In Arthur's case, the remembering of emotional situations was accompanied, innumerable times, by change in
blood pressure and arrhythmia; in Beth's case, the burning sensation
in the joints was constant. With Cecilia, due to the complex phenomena at work, the transformations were less immediate and less
visible. Nevertheless, in this case also, the pain evoked by the paternal image in the region of the surgical scar is proof of the relation
between emotion and physiological change.

It was also clear that the somatic symptoms had strong connections with the parental complexes, both in their origin and in
their development. In almost all cases, the constellation of these
complexes in current situations (evoked by transference or otherwise) happened concomitant with alterations on both the physiological and psychological levels, observable in changes of mood,
emotions, images, fantasies, muscular contractions, inflammations,
pain, arrhythmia, etc.

The stress factor present in numerous research studies is here seen only when current situations mirror a conflict similar to that which gave rise to the primary split. At such moments it is as if the memory of the emotion reappeared in the body. The interaction or non-interaction of a complex with a stressful event could thus explain the controversial results of many studies. That is, a stressful event has a pathological effect only when it strikes a complex. When it does not, it will only cause an emotion that can be consciously elaborated without getting stuck in the body.

At the start of the analytical process, no patient associated the appearance of the disease with emotional conflicts. If instinct is located at the infrared end of the spectrum, and is therefore not accessible to the consciousness, direct contact with it is impossible. Thus, orientation that is direct, or that proceeds through conscious-ness, would be useless. The patients had no access to the organic mechanisms that afflicted them. In the three main cases (Chapter 5), as well as in the vignette cases (Chapter 6), the coenesthetic impres-sions that emerged as the complexes manifested themselves were split from their abstract representations, i.e. the patients did not per-ceive what was taking shape on a psychic plane when their organic symptoms appeared. By working with the psychic contents syn-chronously with their organic symptoms, the patients gradually became conscious of this relation.

This work took place through use of active imagination, sandplay, and expressive and interpretive techniques, which allowed for con-sciousness of the emerging images that referred directly to each patient's organic symptoms. In Arthur, for example, there was the image of the human grenade when he focused his attention on the veins and arteries. In Beth, concentration on the joints led to seeing images of strings (marionettes) and handcuffs that impeded the patient's movements. In Cecilia, there emerged a terrible, gigantic maternal figure that threatened to destroy the patient. By compre-hending these images, among others, it was possible to perceive the nature of the dysfunction in the ego–Self axis.

We could also observe in all the cases presented here how the symptom/symbol mirrored the psychic structure and/or vice versa. In Arthur, the repressed and constricted love life was mirrored syn-chronistically by the cardiac pain and pathology. Or should we say that the constriction in the veins and arteries was mirrored in the love constriction? In Beth, sadness, accumulated resentment and anger were expressed at the organic level by the gradually paralyzing inflammation. The psychic paralysis synchronistically revealed itself in the body as arthritic "paralysis." And in Cecilia, desperation and revolt over a love loss, felt as a death, were portrayed as revolt and the threat of death on a cellular level.

As the images took shape, the symptom's significance was clarified. Because of disturbances present in the primary relationship in almost all cases, it could have been that a split occurred between fantasy life and coenesthetic sensations, preventing the patients from expressing their conflicts verbally or through eidetic images. However, we have proved that none of these patients could be classified as alexithymic. The richness and profusion of images present in all the cases is proof of this.

It is possible that for these patients the primary parental figure that is critical in modulating the infant's psychological and physiological arousal, by not mediating between psyche and body, made the symbolic, transcendent function stay stuck fast in the body, rather than transforming itself into fantasies and images that could be assimilated by the ego. Research in the field of psychoneuroimmunology probably will prove that during critical periods of maturation, environmental and family stress may lead to deregulation of hormone stress level, especially in the brain, resulting in different pathologies.

Our work enhances research data evidencing the effect of stress and emotional expression on the onset and treatment of various diseases. The repression blocking the ability of our patients to express emotions led to the imbedding in the shadow of conflictive contents and complexes associated with bodily sensations and images. Thus, the shadow human grenade is the anger contained for years. In Beth, the sadness and the unconscious anger and resentment present in the shadow are experienced as nodules, which prevent movement. In Cecilia, the needy, injured, abandoned child takes up residence in the body as organic fragility and vulnerability. The psyche induces somatization of those conflictive and traumatic situations that could not be integrated on the conscious plane.

The activity of a compensatory mechanism was also responsible for the meaning of the symptoms. In Arthur, hostility and the attempt to suppress emotional life were compensated by the exuberant manifestation of the heart (stabs). In Beth, hyperactivity was compensated by the blockage of movements, and in Cecilia, the repressed anger exploded in cells out of control. The emergence of the symbol at its concrete, corporal pole forced the patients to confront themselves and their complexes and to correct their one-sided development.

We saw also the quantity and quality of painful information repressed and denied in the patients presented here: repression and denial that, while protecting the organism from unconscious, unbearable, painful information, at the same time reproduce error. The information that cannot be consciously transformed is encapsulated in the complex, producing repetitive pathological symptoms. The disease thus installs itself in the organism and makes it suffer from a lack of coherence on multiple levels. According to Conforti, "the repetition stands as an autonomous event, morphogenetically coded, with an information rich set of directives embedded in each and every system about its developmental trajectory" (Conforti, 1999: 110).

"The repetition creates a number of crucial dynamics in the individual's life" (Conforti, 1999: 112) and may explain certain observable patterns of personality related with some diseases. Probably the somatopsychic archetypal structures give the base for a certain homogeneity of the symbolic body, limiting the organism's possibilities of expression. Arthur at first shows personality traits similar to those denominated in the literature as Type A, while Beth and Cecilia have similarities to Type C. Since all complexes have a universal archetypal basis, perhaps individuals with similar pathological traits have similar somatopsychic structures. That is, similarities in the type of pathology would reflect similarities in dysfunction of the relation between ego, complex, archetype and body, which relation, in turn, has a limited range of representations. Therefore, studies that relate personality traits to diseases may be pointing to a universality in the synchronicity of physiopathological and psychopathological manifestations.

Studies on the symbolism of the body prove this by revealing a relatively limited and universal number of possible projections attributed to each part of the body. For instance, by studying the symbolism of the heart in many different cultures, from pre-history until today, we realize that most myths and images related to this organ refer to a loving and feminine pattern. This archetypical pattern is quite visible in patients with heart disease (Ramos, 1990). The study of the symbolic body thus complements cognitive and empirical studies, in the search for a unified theory.

As a result of all of the above mechanisms, the patients were led to a process that brought them to individuation and to integration of emotional contents. In Arthur, the cardiac suffering led to the perception of amorous suffering and to opening up the love life. In Beth, pain, deformity, and immobility led to her becoming conscious of the denial of desires and the need to enact those desires so that the patient would once again be able to move. And in Cecilia, the wound and the tumors led to her integrating the injured, rejected girl shadow, interrupting a self-destructive process.

We can affirm that in the cases studied (including the vignettes), the organic symptom corresponded to a split in the representation of a complex, where the abstract, psychic part was repressed. The symptom/symbol began to develop automatically and out of control, revealing its complex and unconscious character.

The use of the analytic model in the patients led to the discovery and integration of the abstract pole of the complexes involved. That is, through the analytic model and its psychotherapeutic techniques, it was possible to transduce the symptoms from their organic pole to the abstract, leading their pathological expressions to diminish gradually and bringing about improvement in the patients' general health.

We would, however, like to make it clear here that the significance of a disease is not a datum a priori, but a possible result of the process of reflecting and bringing into consciousness. The obligation to find significance in every disease would lead us to another type of reductionism. The message is rarely clear and there are great variations. Faced with phenomena as complex as health and disease, an absolutist posture would be extremely simplistic. If totality implies health plus sickness, then sickness is an inevitable part of the process of individuation as we encounter it. By so saying, we wish to reinforce once more the idea, described above, that a disease is not necessarily linked to a psychopathological process, but may be indicative of a new symbol. It may or may not be the expression of a new de-integration (personal or in the environment), which needs to be made conscious, always remembering that the more we approach the Self, the more the health–illness polarity may emerge. Creativity, as an instinctive force, may lead as well to health as to disease.

These considerations round out the results obtained here and extend the contribution that the analytic mode may make in this area. The introduction of the concept of disease as symbol resolves the secular psyche–body dichotomy; it also stimulates reflection on redefining the limits of the psychological and the biological, of psychology and medicine: a reflection/redefinition already happening in clinical practice.

Laszlo (2003) in his lecture at the Assisi Conference, when talking about the relationship of psychology, biology and physics, explained the mechanisms that underlie the formation of a malignant cell as an information error: that is, the cancer cell has impoverished information that makes it reproduce itself in a pathological way. What is necessary is to give new information to this cell, and this can be done on different levels. Medication and placebo are two of these; the other is the symbol.

If we understand health as a well-balanced, integrated system, to be healthy is to have a balanced and fluid integration among different systems. A failure in one of them may provoke an imbalance in the whole. The information of an error in the environment, for example, is transduced in the different systems and – according to the level of consciousness of the organism – it may or may not be absorbed in a healthy way.

If we understand disease as a communication breakdown, the question is how to change this process. The interference can be made in any level, or in different levels at the same time. We have to find out which one is most suitable in each case. The use of the symbol as information that may interfere in the dynamic system of the organism is without doubt a possibility that will allow for great advances in interdisciplinary work and research.

What is necessary, therefore, is not merely the production of more scientific data for its own sake, but a theoretical attitude, a language that may serve as a guide for research and clinical practice, keeping the individual as its focus and technology at its service.

We have proved here that the application of the analytic model in different types of disease supplies these theoretical and technical substrata, enhancing various fields of knowledge and widening our comprehension of the complex psyche–body phenomenon.

Appendix: Placebo studies

The extent to which science has come to disregard psychological factors can be seen in its disdainful treatment of both the placebo effect and so-called miracle healings. Though part of our culture from ancient times to the present age, healing through faith (or through belief in the doctor or medicine) has not yet been adequately studied by modern science.

Used frequently in reference to sugar pills, pills that are apparently chemically inert, or any procedure that does not have intrinsic therapeutic value, the word "placebo" literally means "I shall please." It is associated with the idea of pleasure or placating the suffering of the one who takes it (Pei, 1962).

To A.K. Shapiro (1964), a pioneer in placebo research, placebo is any therapeutic procedure, or specific component of a therapeutic procedure, for which there is no objective evidence of a specific activity on the symptom that is being treated.

While there were moments in history in which this type of healing was considered, such as the Romantic period, in the twentieth century the placebo factor was put aside by most research. When it is taken into account, it is interpreted as "spontaneous remission" and never as a result of the influence of the psyche. The concept of transference was restricted to the field of psychological illnesses and was never used effectively to promote healing of organic diseases. Biochemists and doctors, in testing medication (for instance, in the treatment of peptide ulcers), declare that it should be 20 percentage points more effective than the placebo, curing 50 to 60 per cent of the patients (Ornstein and Sobel, 1987). The fact, however, that the placebo has relieved the symptoms of 30 to 40 per cent of the patients goes by, generally, unheeded, drawing no further reflections, and confirms the resistance still met with today. Yet, what wonderful "drug" is this that cures 30 to 40 per cent of the patients with "nothing"?

More scientific studies, in which neither the patients nor the doctors know they are using the placebo, have shown that 35 per cent of the patients within a wide range of postsurgical pains have obtained significant relief with the placebo. In some studies pain relief has reached 50 per cent. More highly controlled research has discovered consistently that around one third of the patients attain more than 50 per cent relief (Evans, 1985).

Evans (1985), in his experimental studies, concluded that the effectiveness of the placebo, when compared with standard dosages of different analgesic drugs, in double-blind circumstances, seems to be relatively constant and proportional to the apparent effectiveness of the active analgesic agent. In an analysis of various studies, Evans concluded that the placebo is 55 to 60 per cent as effective as active medication, regardless of its potency.

As such, while the placebo effect is still rejected by many as a "disturbing factor," incomprehensible and insignificant, to others it has been worthy of attention as a fundamental element in the healing process. Its study allows a new perspective in understanding the psyche–body communication and how the psyche can bring about biochemical changes, essential in the mobilization of body defenses.

If we start giving the placebo its due attention, we will very likely discover it to be a powerful therapeutic instrument whose effects are an integral part of daily clinical practice (Straus and von Ammon Cavanaugh, 1996). A.K. Shapiro (1960) has frequently been cited as having said that the history of medical treatment can be characterized as the history of the placebo effect, since until recently all medication was placebo (Ornstein and Sobel, 1987).

Throughout the ages there have been a variety of highly improbable medications, such as animal excrement, mummy powder, bat blood, dried snake, toad sperm, and so on. Despite (or perhaps because of) their improbability, these potions have made people feel better. Rossi (1986) observes in such cases that there must be some reason for the healing of the sick person. The first possible reason is that these unlikely medications contain some physiologically active ingredient. The second is that most diseases end of their own accord. They follow their natural cycle, with or without medical intervention. As most people consult the doctor at their worst, when they get better, the cure is attributed to the treatment and not to the natural cycle of the disease.

Another explanation for the unexpected recovery is that perhaps it is not the medication that cures, but rather the belief in the medication and in the healer sets off some powerful mechanism of self-healing within the body (Rossi, 1986).

As such, we may consider the placebo as a tangible symbol that something is being done to help the patient. It triggers a network of powerful personal and cultural expectations that the patient will get better. In our society, with its belief in a better life through technology and chemistry, what could be better than a pill, an injection or even a surgical procedure? These meet our needs for something tangible, visible, to which may be attributed a cure.

According to Ornstein and Sobel (1987), there are some myths about placebos that must be dispelled.

1 Placebos are physiologically inert and therefore work only for psychological symptoms. There is clear evidence that this point of view is fallacious. Henry Beecher, of Harvard Medical School, reviewed a great number of studies and discovered that, on average, one-third of those who received placebos reported relief from their symptoms (Beecher, 1955). The symptoms included pain in the post-surgical wound, nausea, headache, cough, anxiety and other problems. Even knowing that the pain experience is subjective, we could not affirm that post-surgical pain is not organic.

2 The placebo effect is very weak. On the contrary, there are at least some indications that the placebo effect is strong enough to surpass the known pharmacological activity of a drug (Wolf, 1950).

3 Placebos are always good. In fact, not all placebo effects are positive and therapeutic, and a negative effect is known as nocebo (from the Latin "I shall harm"). When the patient attaches negative meanings and emotions to a treatment, a range of disagreeable symptoms can arise, including palpitations, dizziness, headaches, diarrhea, nausea and skin lesions (Frank, 1975; Margo, 1999, Papakostas and Daras, 2001).

But what is it that makes a placebo function or not? It seems, according to Sobel (1990), that some people have a greater response to placebos than others, though there is as yet no data to determine whether a personality trait is involved. Most likely, the same person may respond to the placebo under certain circumstances and not others, for motivations or symptom meanings brought by a person to a specific situation have greater weight than personality traits, though the two may interact. This observation was confirmed in the laboratory, where a study under strict control of variables showed that motivation, rather than expectation, is the predominant factor in perceiving a change in the symptom (Jensen and Karoly, 1991).

Our beliefs in the nature of the treatment and its physical characteristics can also affect the placebo effect. It seems that famous brands and doctors, the doctor's enthusiasm and confidence in the effect of the drug, and injections as opposed to pills, increase the placebo effect (Sobel, 1990). The message given with any treatment can also influence the speed with which it gets results. In a study of 30 patients in relaxation training to lower blood pressure, half were told that their pressure would lower immediately after a session, while others were told that this would happen only after the third session. Those who expected an immediate response showed a seven times greater reduction of the systolic arterial pressure compared to that of the other group (Agras et al., 1982).

According to Benson and Friedman (1996), the placebo effect yields beneficial clinical results in 60–90 per cent of diseases, including angina pectoris, bronchial asthma, herpes simplex and duodenal ulcer. Double-blind randomized controlled trials have shown that placebos can have healing effects in such diverse conditions as angina pectoris (Benson and McCallie, 1979), epilepsy (UK Gabapentin Study Group, 1990), pain treatment (Turner et al., 1994) and cancer (Downer et al., 1994).

Research (Rossi, 1986; Benson and Friedman, 1996) has revealed that the placebo response is a healing factor in various diseases involving:

1   the immune system – cancer, warts, herpes simplex, common cold, fever, vaccines, bronchial asthma, multiple sclerosis and rheumatoid arthritis
2   the autonomic nervous system – hypertension, pupillary dilatation, blood cell count, headaches, epilepsy and stress
3   the endocrine system – diabetes, ulcers, gastric secretion and motility, colitis and menstrual pain
4   the circulatory system – angina pectoris, congestive heart failure, and mortality in coronary artery disease.

It is also a healing factor in surgical or psychological treatments, such as conditioning (systematic desensitization), and perhaps in all types of psychotherapy (Shapiro and Morris, 1978; Rossi, 1986; Papakostas and Daras, 2001). Although some symptoms seem more prone to the influence of placebos than others, it appears that no system is immune to the placebo effect. It is thus impossible, for instance, for a doctor to use a placebo to distinguish between psychogenic pain and pain due to organic causes.

The implication of these discoveries is that there is a placebo response of 55 per cent in many healing procedures. Such a degree of consistent placebo response suggests that an underlying common mechanism or process is responsible for mind–body communication and cure, independent of the problem, symptom or disease.

The mechanism by which belief in the placebo is translated into positive physiological changes is still unknown. There is evidence that links placebo anesthesia to the liberation of endorphins. The more the physiology of the placebo is understood, the more we will be able to elaborate therapeutic interventions that trigger these intricate healing systems.

While the placebo effect provides evidence that there are certain self-healing mechanisms within us, intrinsic healing systems that can be mobilized if given the appropriate environmental and situational signs, it is also one of the best proofs of the psyche–body phenomenon.

Up to now, we have mobilized these dynamics in an unconscious way, through magic, suggestion, beliefs. Our difficulty in dealing with the non-measurable, the intangible, leads us to attribute to the external and material the power that belongs to the psyche. The pill is necessary in a culture that feels uncomfortable with the "invisible" and would rather think that any internal effect must have an external cause. The placebo can transform the "desire to live" into a physical reality, just as emotional conflict, expressing itself somatically, does so. That is, finding it hard to express a conflict on the abstract level, the organism "materializes" it, making it thus more "accessible," more "visible."

To sum up, these studies show how a symbol can act on a body, triggering a symptom or helping the healing process. The placebo intermediates the psyche's activity over matter, and, as such, is a concrete, facilitating symbol in the psyche–body phenomenon.

The challenge that follows is to develop alternative means by which to begin to understand the dynamic mechanisms of these intrinsic systems and learn to mobilize them in healing, since they certainly participate actively in forming the disease.

Notes

Introduction

1   Many of the ideas developed here approximate those of Mara Sidoli (2000). As Sidoli was probably unaware of my hypothesis, which had been published only in Portuguese, the similarity of ideas is surprising and supports the model described here. I therefore recommend her book as complementary reading to this one.

Chapter 1

1   Alexithymia: from the Greek *alexo*, to separate, expel; and *thymos*, soul, desire; literally, drawing away from desire or from the soul.

Chapter 2

1   For a more detailed discussion of this subject I recommend Jacoby (1999).

Chapter 3

1   For a detailed study on symbolism I recommend Kast (1992).

Chapter 5

1   Myocardial infarction is gross necrosis of the myocardium as a result of interruption of the blood supply to the area; it is almost always caused by atherosclerosis of the coronary arteries, upon which coronary thrombosis is usually superimposed. The word "infarct" comes from the Latin *infarcire* meaning "to plug up or cram."

2   Rheumatoid arthritis is usually a chronic disease and is considered an autoimmune disease. It is a disorder of connective tissue, characterized by inflammation, degeneration, pain, stiffness, swelling, and sometimes destruction of joints.

3   Melanoma is a skin tumor containing dark pigment and with high malignancy that starts in melanocytes of normal skin or moles and metastasizes rapidly and widely.

4   A mammary cyst is an abnormal sac in the mammary gland, filled with a fluid or semisolid and enclosed in a membrane.

Chapter 6

1   Acne rosacea is acne involving the skin of the nose, forehead, and cheeks and is characterized by congestion, flushing, telangiectasia, and marked nodular swelling of tissues, especially of the nose; also called "rosacea."
2   Sandplay is a non-verbal Jungian technique developed by Dora Kalf in the 1930s that uses sand and water in a tray in which toys or miniatures are placed. H. Friedman and R.R. Mitchell are working on the relationship of sandplay and the effects of trauma on the brain (lecture given at Pontificia Universidade Catolica de São Paulo, 26 September 2003).
3   Fecaloma is an accumulation of inspissated feces formed in the rectum or distal colon with the appearance of an abdominal tumor.
4   Reynaud's syndrome is a disorder of blood circulation in the fingers and toes that is aggravated by exposure to the cold. The disorder is sometimes called white finger, wax finger or dead finger. Why it occurs is not well understood. Normally, the body conserves heat by reducing blood circulation to the extremities, particularly the hands and feet. This response uses a complex system of nerves and muscles to control blood flow through the smallest blood vessels in the skin. In people with Reynaud's syndrome, this control system becomes too sensitive to cold and greatly reduces blood flow in the fingers.
5   Pelvic inflammatory disease is an infection of the female reproductive tract that results especially from microorganisms transmitted during sexual intercourse. It is marked by lower abdominal pain and abnormal vaginal discharge.
6   Migraine is a condition that is marked by recurrent, usually unilateral, severe headache, often accompanied by nausea and vomiting. It is of uncertain origin, though attacks appear to be precipitated by dilatation of intracranial blood vessels.
7   Miscarriage is a spontaneous expulsion of a human fetus before it is viable, especially between the 12th and 28th weeks of gestation.

Bibliography

Agras, W.S., Horne, M. and Taylor, C.B. (1982) "Expectation and blood-pressure lowering effect of relaxation", *Psychosomatic Medicine*, **44**: 389–395.

Albrecht, A. (1979) *Satsanga – Contos da India*, São Paulo: Nova Acrópole.

Alexander, F. (1923/1989) *Medicina Psicossomática*, Porto Alegre, Brazil: Editora Artes Médicas Sul.

Almada, S., Zonderman, A., Shekelle, R., Dyer, A., Daviglus, M., Costa, P. and Stamler, J. (1991) "Neuroticism, cynicism and risk of death in middle-aged men: The Western Electric Study", *Psychosomatic Medicine*, **53**: 165–175.

Ananth, J. and Burnstein, M. (1977) "Cancer: less common in psychiatric patients?" *Psychosomatics*, **18**, 2: 44–46.

Andersen, B.L., Farrar, W.B., Golden-Kreutz, D., Kutz, L.A., MacCallum, R., Courtney, M.E. and Glaser, R. (1998) "Stress and immune responses after surgical treatment for regional breast cancer", *Journal of the National Cancer Institute*, **90**, 1: 30–36.

Anderson, K., Bradley, L., Young, L., McDaniel, L. and Wise, C. (1985) "Rheumatoid arthritis: review of psychological factors related to etiology, effects, and treatment", *Psychological Bulletin*, **98**: 358–387.

Appels, A. (1997) "Depression and coronary heart disease: observations and questions", *Journal of Psychosomatic Research*, **43**, 5: 443–452.

Atchison, M. and Condon, J. (1993) "Hostility and anger measures in coronary heart disease", *The Australian and New Zealand Journal of Psychiatry*, **27**, 3: 436–442.

Barefoot, J.C., Larsen, S., von der Lieth, L. and Schroll, M. (1995) "Hostility, incidence of acute myocardial infarction, and mortality in a sample of older Danish men and women", *American Journal of Epidemiology*, **142**, 5: 477–484.

Beecher, H.K. (1955) "The powerful placebo", *Journal of the American Medical Association*, **159**: 1602–1606.

Benson, H. and Friedman, R. (1996) "Harnessing the power of the placebo effect and renaming it 'remembered wellness' ", *Annual Review of Medicine*, **47**: 193–199.

Benson, H. and McCallie, D.P. Jr (1979) "Angina pectoris and the placebo effect", *The New England Journal of Medicine*, **300**, 25: 1424–1429.

Bieliauskas, L. and Garron, D. (1982) "Psychological depression and cancer", *General Hospital Psychiatry*, **4**: 187–195.

Bleiker, E.M., van der Ploeg, H.M., Hendriks, J.H. and Ader, H.J. (1996) "Personality factors and breast cancer development: a prospective longitudinal study", *Journal of the National Cancer Institute*, **88**, 20: 1478–1482.

Bradley, L., Young, L., Anderson, K., Turner, R., Agudelo, C., McDaniel, L., Pisko, E., Semble, E. and Morgan, T. (1987) "Effects of psychological therapy on pain behaviour of rheumatoid arthritis patients", *Arthritis and Rheumatism*, **30**: 1105–1114.

Brown, T.M. (1990) "Cartesian dualism and psychosomatics", *Psychosomatics*, **30**, 3: 213–221.

Byington, C.A. (1988) *Dimensões Simbólicas da Personalidade*, São Paulo: Ática.

Cabral, M., Giglio, J. and Stangenhaus, G. (1988) "A relação trabalho-lazer em pacientes acometidos de artrite reumatóide", *Jornal Brasileiro de Psiquiatria*, **6**: 303–308.

Campbell, J. (1990) *O Poder do Mito*, São Paulo: Editora Palas Athena.

Canguilhem, G. (1978) *O Normal e o Patológico*, Rio de Janeiro: Forense Universitária.

Capra, F. (1982) *The Turning Point*, New York: Simon and Schuster.

Carette, S., Surtees, P.G., Wainwright, N.W., Khaw, K.T., Symmons, D.P. and Silman, A.J. (2000) "The role of life events and childhood experiences in the development of rheumatoid arthritis", *The Journal of Rheumatology*, **27**, 9: 2123–2130.

Carney, R., Freedland, K. and Jaffe, A. (1990) "Insomnia and depression prior to myocardial infarction", *Psychosomatic Medicine*, **52**: 603–609.

Castiel, L.D. (1991) "Psicossomática e eficácia: além do princípio do placebo", *Jornal Brasileiro de Psiquiatria*, **40**, 5: 267–272.

Chaput, L.A., Adams, S.H., Simon, J.A., Blumenthal, R.S., Vittinghoff, E., Lin, F., Loh, E. and Matthews, K.A. (2002) "Hostility predicts recurrent events among postmenopausal women with coronary heart disease", *American Journal of Epidemiology*, **156**, 12: 1092–1099.

Chesney, M., Ekman, P., Friesen, W., Black, G. and Hecker, M. (1990) "Type A behavior pattern: facial behavior and speech components", *Psychosomatic Medicine*, **53**: 307–319.

Cohen, M., Dembling, B. and Schorling, J. (2002) "The association between schizophrenia and cancer: a population-based mortality study", *Schizophrenia Research*, **57**, 2–3: 139–146.

Cohen, S. (1990) "Social support and physical illness", *Advances*, **7**, 1: 35–48.

Cohen, S. and Syme, S.L. (eds) (1985) *Social Support and Health*, New York: Academic Press.

Conforti, M. (1999) *Field, Form and Fate*, New Orleans: Spring Journal Books.

Conger, J.P. (1988) *Jung and Reich: The Body as Shadow*, Berkeley, CA: North Atlantic Books.

Costa, P. Jr, Krantz, D., Blumenthal, J., Furberg, C., Rosenman, R. and Shekelle, R. (1987) "Task force 2: psychological risk factors in coronary artery disease", *Circulation*, **276**, suppl.: 1145–1149.

Craig, T.J. and Lin, S.P. (1981) "Cancer and mental illness", *Comprehensive Psychiatry*, **22**, 4: 404–410.

Dalton, S.O., Boesen, E.H., Ross, L., Schapiro, I.R. and Johansen, C. (2002) "Mind and cancer: do psychological factors cause cancer?", *European Journal of Cancer*, **38**, 10: 1313–1323.

Dattore, P.J., Shontz, F.C. and Coyne, L. (1980) "Premorbid personality differentiation of cancer and non cancer groups: a test of the hypothesis of cancer proneness", *Journal of Consulting and Clinical Psychology*, **48**, 3: 388–394.

Dembroski, T., MacDougall, J., Williams, R., Haney, T. and Blumenthal, J. (1985) "Components of type A hostility, and anger-In", *Psychosomatic Medicine*, **47**: 219–233.

Derogatis, L.R., Abeloff, M. and Melisaratos, N. (1979) "Psychological coping mechanisms and survival time in metastatic breast cancer", *Journal of the American Medical Association*, **242**: 1504–1508.

Descartes, R. (1955) "The passions of the soul", in E.S. Haldane (ed.) *The Philosophical Works*, vol. 1, New York: Dover.

—— (1971) "Discourse on method XI, 120", in J.M. Morus (ed.) *Descartes Dictionary*, New York: Philosophical Library.

—— (1988) "Meditação Sexta. Da Existência das Coisas Materiais e da Distinção real entre a Alma e o Corpo do Homem", in J. Guinsburg and B. Prado (eds) *Meditações*, São Paulo: Nova Cultural.

Deutsch, F. (1922) "Der gesunde und der kranke korper in psychoanalytischer betrachtung", *Int. Zeit. Psa*, **8**: 290.

Doran, M.F., Pond, G.R., Crowson, C.S., O'Fallon, W.M., and Gabriel, S.E. (2002) "Trends in incidence and mortality in rheumatoid arthritis in Rochester, Minnesota, over a forty-year period", *Arthritis and Rheumatism*, **46**, 3: 625–631.

Downer, S.M., Cody, M.M., McCluskey, P., Wilson, P.D., Arnott, S.J., Lister, T.A. and Slevin, M.L. (1994) "Pursuit and practice of complementary therapies by cancer patients receiving conventional treatment", *British Medical Journal*, **309**, 6947: 86–89.

Dunbar, H. (1935) *Emotions and Bodily Changes: A Survey of Literature on Psychosomatic Interrelationships 1910–1933*, New York: Columbia University Press.

Eaton, W.W., Hayward, C. and Ram, R. (1992) "Schizophrenia and rheumatoid arthritis: a review", *Schizophrenia Research*, **6**: 182–192.

The Editors (1939) "Editorial", *Psychosomatic Medicine*, **1**: 3–5.

Engebretson, T. and Matthews, K. (1992) "Dimensions of hostility in men, women, and boys: relationships to personality and cardiovascular responses to stress", *Psychosomatic Medicine*, **54**: 311–323.

Esterling, B., Antoni, M., Kumar, M. and Schneiderman, N. (1990) "Emotional repression, stress disclosure responses, and Epstein-Barr viral capsid antigen titers", *Psychosomatic Medicine*, **52**: 397–410.

Evans, F. (1985) "Expectancy, therapeutic instructions, and the placebo response", in L. White and G. Schwartz (eds) *Placebo: Theory, Reseach, and Mechanisms*, New York: Guilford Press.

Everson, S.A., Goldberg, D.E., Kaplan, G.A., Cohen, R.D., Pukkala, E., Tuomilehto, J. and Salonen, J.T. (1996) "Hopelessness and risk of mortality and incidence of myocardial infarction and cancer", *Psychosomatic Medicine*, **58**: 113–121.

Fabrega, H. Jr (1990) "The concept of somatization as a cultural and historical product of western medicine", *Psychosomatic Medicine*, **52**, 6: 653–672.

Faragher, E.B. and Cooper, C.L. (1990) "Type A stress prone behaviour and breast cancer", *Psychological Medicine*, **20**, 3: 663–670.

Felitti, V.J., Anda, R.F., Nordenberg, D., Williamson, D.F., Spitz, A.M., Edwards, V., Koss, M.P. and Marks, J.S. (1998) "Relationship of childhood abuse and household dysfunction to many of the leading causes of death in adults. The Adverse Childhood Experiences (ACE) Study", *American Journal of Preventive Medicine*, **14**, 4: 245–258.

Ferguson, M. (1980) *The Aquarian Conspiracy*, Los Angeles: J.P. Tarcher.

Fordham, M. (1957) *New Developments in Analytical Psychology*, London: Routledge & Kegan Paul.

Foss, L. and Rothenberg, K. (1987) *The Second Medical Revolution. From Biomedicine to Informedicine*, Boston: Shambala.

Frank, J.D. (1975) "The faith that heals", *The Johns Hopkins Medical Journal*, **137**: 127–131.

Frasure-Smith, N., Lespérance, F., Juneau, M., Talajic, M. and Bourassa, M.G. (1999) "Gender, depression, and one-year prognosis after myocardial infarction", *Psychosomatic Medicine*, **61**, 1: 26–37.

Freud, S. (1891/1954) *On Aphasia: A Critical Study*, New York: International Universities Press.

—— (1895/1966) *Project for a scientific psychology*. In E. Jones (ed.) & J. Strachey (trans.) *The Standard Edition of the Complete Psychological Works of Sigmund Freud*, Vol. 1. London: Hogarth Press.

Friedman, M. and Rosenman, R. (1974) *Type A Behavior and Your Heart*, New York: Alfred A. Knopf.

Fuller, B. (1963) *Operating Manual for Spaceship Earth*. http: //www.bfi.org/ operating_manual.htm (accessed 7 January 2004).

Funk and Wagnalls (1950) *New College Standard Dictionary*, New York: Funk & Wagnalls.

Gallacher, J.E., Yarnell, J.W., Sweetnam, P.M., Elwood, P.C. and Stansfeld, S.A. (1999) "Anger and incident heart disease in the Caerphilly study", *Psychosomatic Medicine*, **61**, 4: 446–453.

Gallo, J.J., Armenian, H.K., Ford, D.E., Eaton, W.W. and Khachaturian, A.S. (2000) "Major depression and cancer: the 13-year follow-up of the Baltimore epidemiologic catchment area sample (United States)", *Cancer Causes & Control*, **11**, 8: 751–758.

Gallo, L.C., Troxel, W.M., Matthews, K.A. and Kuller, L.H. (2003) "Marital status and quality in middle-aged women: associations with levels and trajectories of cardiovascular risk factors", *Health Psychology*, **22**, 5: 453–463.

Gerin, W., Pieper, C., Levy, R. and Pickering, T. (1992) "Social support in social interaction: a moderator of cardiovascular reactivity", *Psychosomatic Medicine*, **54**: 324–336.

Geyer, S. (1991) "Life events prior to manifestation of breast cancer: a limited prospective study covering eight years before diagnosis", *Journal of Psychosomatic Research*, **35**, 2–3: 355–363.

Geyer, S. (1993) "Life events, chronic difficulties and vulnerability factors preceding breast cancer", *Journal of Psychosomatic Research*, **37**, 12: 1545–1555.

Gloria, F., Meaney, E., Rivera, J.M., Robles, A. and Vela, A. (1996) "The hostility complex and myocardial infarct" (in Spanish), *Archivos del Instituto de Cardiologia de Mexico*, **66**, 2: 138–142.

Goldstein, D. and Antoni, M. (1989) "The distribution of repressive coping styles among non-metastatic breast cancer patients as compared to non-cancer controls", *Psychology and Health*, **3**: 245–258.

Gore, S. (1978) "The effect of social support in moderating the health consequences of unemployment", *Journal of Health and Social Behavior*, **19**: 157–165.

Greer, S. and Morris, T. (1975) "Psychological attributes of women who develop breast cancer: a controlled study", *Journal of Psychosomatic Research*, **19**: 147–153.

Greer, S., Morris, T. and Pettingale, K. (1979) "Psychological response to breast cancer: effect on outcome", *Lancet*, **2**: 785–787.

Groddeck, G. (1949) *The Book of the It*, New York: Vintage Books.

Groddeck, G. (1992) *Estudos Psicanalíticos sobre Psicossomática*, São Paulo: Editora Perspectiva.

Gulbinat, W., Dupont, A., Jablensky, A., Jensen, O.M., Marsella, A., Nakane, Y. and Sartorius, N. (1992) "Cancer incidence of schizophrenic patients. Results of record linkage studies in three countries", *British Journal of Psychiatry*, **18**, suppl.: 75–83.

Gusdorf, G. (1984) *L'Homme Romantique*, Paris: Payot.

Hahn, R. and Petitti, D. (1988) "Minnesota Multiphasic Personality Inventory: rated depression and the incidence of breast cancer", *Cancer*, **61**: 845–848.

Harris, A.E. (1988) "Physical disease and schizophrenia", *Schizophrenia Bulletin*, **14**, 1: 85–96.

Haynal, A. and Pasini, W. (1983) *Manual de Medicina Psicossomática*, São Paulo: Editora Masson.

Hecker, M.H., Chesney, M.A., Black, G.W. and Frautschi, N. (1988) "Coronary-prone behaviors in the Western Collaborative Group Study", *Psychosomatic Medicine*, **50**, 2: 153–164.

Heidbreder, E. (1964) *Psicologias del Siglo XX*, Buenos Aires: Editorial Paidos.

Hislop, T., Waxler, N. and Coldman, A. (1987) "The prognostic significance of psychosocial factors in women with breast cancer", *Journal of Chronic Disease*, **40**: 729–735.

Horning-Rohan, M. and Locke, S. (1985) *Psychological and Behavioral Treatments for Disorders of the Heart and Blood Vessels*, New York: Institute for the Advancement of Health.

Horsten, M., Ericson, M., Perski, A., Wamala, S.P., Schenck-Gustafsson, K. and Orth-Gomér, K. (1999) "Psychosocial factors and heart rate variability in healthy women", *Psychosomatic Medicine*, **61**, 1: 49–57.

Hussar, A.E. (1996) "Leading causes of death in institutionalized chronic schizophrenic patients: a study of 1,275 autopsy protocols", *The Journal of Nervous and Mental Disease*, **142**, 1: 45–57.

Irwin, M., Smith, T. and Gillin, J. (1992) "Electroencephalographic sleep and natural killer activity in depressed patients and control subjects", *Psychosomatic Medicine*, **54**: 10–21.

Jacobs, J.R. and Bovasso, G.B. (2000) "Early and chronic stress and their relation to breast cancer", *Psychological Medicine*, **30**, 3: 669–678.

Jacoby, M. (1999) *Jungian Psychotherapy and Contemporary Infant Research*, London: Routledge.

Jamner, L., Shapiro, D., Goldstein, I. and Hug, R. (1991) "Ambulatory blood pressure and heart rate in paramedics: effects of cynical hostility and defensiveness", *Psychosomatic Medicine*, **53**: 393–406.

Jensen, M. and Karoly, P. (1991) "Motivation and expectancy in symptom perception: a laboratory study of the placebo effect", *Psychosomatic Medicine*, **53**: 144–152.

Jones, D.R., Goldblatt, P.O. and Leon, D.A. (1984) "Bereavement and cancer: some data on deaths of spouses from the longitudinal study of Office of Population Censuses and Surveys", *British Medical Journal (Clinical Research edn)*, **289**, 6443: 461–464.

Jorgensen, R.S., Frankowski, J.J., Lantinga, L.J., Phadke, K., Sprafkin, R.P. and Abdul-Karim, K.W. (2001) "Defensive hostility and coronary heart disease: a preliminary investigation of male veterans", *Psychosomatic Medicine*, **63**, 3: 463–469.

Jung, C.G. (1953/1992) *The Collected Works of Carl G. Jung* (Bollingen Series XX) (trans. R.F.C. Hull; eds H. Read, M. Fordham, G. Adler and W. Mc Guire), London: Routledge & Kegan Paul.

—— (1953) *Two Essays on Analytical Psychology*, Collected Works: 7.

—— (1968) *Psychology and Alchemy*, Collected Works: 12.

—— (1970) *Symbols of Transformation*, Collected Works: 5.

—— (1971) *Psychological Types*, Collected Works: 6.

—— (1972) *The Structure and Dynamics of the Psyche*, Collected Works: 8.

—— (1973) *Experimental Researches*, Collected Works: 2.

—— (1974) *Aion*, Collected Works: 9 (II).

—— (1975) *The Archetypes and the Collective Unconscious*, Collected Works: 9 (I).

—— (1988) *Nietzsche's Zarathustra*, Bollingen Series XCIX, vol. 1, Princeton, NJ: Princeton University Press.

Kamarck, T., Manuck, S. and Jennings, R. (1990) "Social support reduces cardiovascular reactivity to psychological challenge: a laboratory model", *Psychosomatic Medicine*, **52**: 42–58.

Kast, V. (1992) *The Dynamics of Symbols: Fundamentals of Jungian Psychotherapy*, New York: International Publishing Corporation.

Kaufmann, M.W., Fitzgibbons, J.P., Sussman, E.J., Reed, J.F. III, Einfalt, J.M., Rodgers, J.K. and Fricchione, G.L. (1999) "Relation between myocardial infarction, depression, hostility, and death", *American Heart Journal*, **138**, 3, pt 1: 549–554.

Kidd, S.M. (2002) *The Secret Life of Bees*, New York: Viking Press.

Kiecolt-Glaser, J., Garner, W., Apeicher, C., Penn, G. and Glaser, R. (1984) "Psychosocial modifiers of immunocompetence in medical students", *Psychosomatic Medicine*, **46**: 7–14.

Kiecolt-Glaser, J., Glaser, R., Strain, E., Stout, J., Holliday, J. and Speicher, C. (1986) "Modulation of cellular immunity in medical students", *Journal of Behavioral Medicine*, **9**: 5–21.

King, K.B. (1997) "Psychologic and social aspects of cardiovascular disease", *Annals of Behavioral Medicine*, **19**, 3: 264–270.

Knapp, P. (1980) "Free association as a biopsychosocial probe", *Psychosomatic Medicine*, **42**: 197–219.

Knapp, P., Levy, E., Giorgi, R., Black, P., Fox, B. and Heeren, T. (1992) "Short-term immunological effects of induced emotion", *Psychosomatic Medicine*, **54**: 133–148.

Kohler, W. (1947) *Gestalt Psychology*, New York: Mentor.

Kornfeld, D.S. (1990) "The American Psychosomatic Society: why?" *Psychosomatic Medicine*, **52**, 4: 481–495.

Kvikstad, A. and Vatten, L.J. (1996) "Risk and prognosis of cancer in middle-aged women who have experienced the death of a child", *International Journal of Cancer*, **67**, 2: 165–169.

Kvikstad, A., Vatten, L.J., Tretli, S. and Kvinnsland, S. (1994) "Death of a husband or marital divorce related to risk of breast cancer in middle-aged women. A nested case–control study among Norwegian women born 1935–1954", *European Journal of Cancer*, **30A**, 4: 473–477.

Lahad, A., Heckbert, S.R., Koepsell, T.D., Psaty, B.M. and Patrick, D.L. (1997) "Hostility, aggression and the risk of nonfatal myocardial infarction in postmenopausal women", *Journal of Psychosomatic Research*, **43**, 2: 183–195.

Laszlo, E. (1993) *The Creative Cosmos. A Unified Science of Matter, Life and Mind*, Edinburgh: Floris.

Laszlo, E. (2003) Lecture at Assisi Conference, Italy. Organized by Michael Conforti, founder and director of the Assisi Foundation.

Latman, N.S. and Walls, R. (1996) "Personality and stress: an exploratory comparison of rheumatoid arthritis and osteoarthritis", *Archives of Physical Medicine and Rehabilitation*, **77**, 8: 796–800.

LeShan, L. (1992) "Creating a climate for self-healing: the principles of modern psychosomatic medicine", *Advances*, **8**, 4: 20–27.

Lespérance, F., Frasure-Smith, N. and Talajic, M. (1996) "Major depression before and after myocardial infarction: its nature and consequences", *Psychosomatic Medicine*, **58**, 2: 99–110.

Levav, I., Kohn, R., Iscovich, J., Abramson, J.H., Tsai, W.Y. and Vigdorovich, D. (2000) "Cancer incidence and survival following bereavement", *American Journal of Public Health*, **90**, 10: 1601–1607.

Lindberg, N.E., Lindberg, E., Theorell, T. and Larsson, G. (1996) "Psychotherapy in rheumatoid arthritis – a parallel-process study of psychic state and course of rheumatic disease", *Zeitschrift für Rheumatologie*, **55**, 1: 28–39.

Lipowski, Z.J. (1984) "What does the word 'psychosomatic' really mean? A historical and semantic inquiry", *Psychosomatic Medicine*, **46**, 2: 153–171.

Loberiza, F.R. Jr, Rizzo, J.D., Bredeson, C.N., Antin, J.H., Horowitz, M.M., Weeks, J.C. and Lee, S.J. (2002) "Association of depressive syndrome and early deaths among patients after stem-cell transplantation for malignant diseases", *Journal of Clinical Oncology*, **20**, 8: 2118–2126.

Lynch, J.J. (1977) *The Broken Heart: The Medical Consequences of Loneliness*, New York: Basic Books.

Lynch, J.J. (1985) *The Language of the Heart: The Human Body in Dialogue*, New York: Basic Books.

McDougall, J. (1986) *Theaters of the Mind*, New York: Basic Books.

McDougall, J. (1989) *Theaters of the Body*, New York: Norton Professional.

McKenna, M.C., Zevon, M.A., Corn, B. and Rounds, J. (1999) "Psychosocial factors and the development of breast cancer: a meta-analysis", *Health Psychology*, **18**, 5: 520–531.

Maddison, D. and Viola, A. (1968) "The health of widows in the year following bereavement", *Journal of Psychosomatic Research*, **12**: 297–306.

Marcenaro, M., Prete, C., Badini, A., Sulli, A., Magi, E. and Cutolo, M. (1999) "Rheumatoid arthritis, personality, stress response style, and coping with illness. A preliminary survey", *Annals of the New York Academy of Sciences*, **876**: 419–425.

Margetts, E.L. (1950) "The early history of the word 'psychosomatic' ", *Canadian Medical Association Journal*, **63**: 402–404.

Margo, C.E. (1999) "The placebo effect", *Survey of Ophthalmology*, **44**, 1: 31–44.

Martikainen, P. and Valkonen, T. (1996) Mortality after the death of a spouse: rates and causes of death in a large Finnish cohort, *American Journal of Public Health*, **86**, 8, pt 1: 1087–1093.

Martins, J. and Bicudo, M.A. (1989) *A Pesquisa Qualitativa em Psicologia Educativa*, São Paulo: EDUC e Editora Moraes.

Marty, P. (1990) *A Psicossomática do Adulto*, Porto Alegre, Brazil: Artes Médicas Sul.

Marty, P., M'Uzan, M. de and David, C. (1963) *L'Investigation Psychosomatique*, Paris: Presses Universitaires de France.

Matthews, K.A. and Gump, B.B. (2002) "Chronic work stress and marital dissolution increase risk of posttrial mortality in men from the Multiple Risk Factor Intervention Trial", *Archives of Internal Medicine*, **162**, 3: 309–315.

Mauceri, J. (1986) *The Great Break*, New York: Pulse.

Meesters, C.M. and Smulders, J. (1994) "Hostility and myocardial infarction in men", *Journal of Psychosomatic Research*, **38**, 7: 727–734.

Meir, C.A. (1986) *Soul and Body*, San Francisco: The Lapis Press.

Mello Filho, J. *et al.* (1992) *Psicossomática Hoje*, Porto Alegre, Brazil Editora Artes Médicas Sul.

Mindell, A. (1982) *Dreambody*, Santa Monica, CA: Sigo Press.

Mindell, A. (1985) *Working with the Dreaming Body*, Boston: Routledge & Kegan Paul.

Moos, R. (1964) "Personality factors associated with rheumatoid arthritis: a review", *Journal of Chronic Disease*, **17**: 41–55.

Mortensen, P.B. (1989) "The incidence of cancer in schizophrenic patients", *Journal of Epidemiology and Community Health*, **43**, 1: 43–47.

Mortensen, P.B. (1994) "The occurrence of cancer in schizophrenic patients", *Schizophrenia Research*, **12**: 185–194.

Myers, S. and Benson, H. (1992) "Psychological factors in healing: a new perspective on an old debate", *Behavioral Medicine*, **18**, 1: 5–10.

Naliboff, B., Benton, D., Solomon, G., Morley, J., Fahey, J., Bloom, E., Makinodan, T. and Gilmore, S. (1991) "Immunological changes in young and old adults during brief laboratory stress", *Psychosomatic Medicine*, **53**: 121–132.

Neumann, E. (1973) *The Origins and History of Consciousness*, Princeton, NJ: Princeton University Press.

Niaura, R., Todaro, J.F., Stroud, L., Spiro, A. III., Ward, K.D. and Weiss, S. (2002) "Hostility, the metabolic syndrome, and incident coronary heart disease", *Health Psychology*, **21**, 6: 588–593.

Odegard, O. (1967) "Mortality in Norwegian psychiatric hospitals 1950–1962", *Acta Genetica et Statistica Medica*, **17**, 1: 137–153.

O'Leary, A. (1990) "Stress, emotion, and human immune function", *Psychological Bulletin*, **108**, 3: 363–382.

Ornstein, R. and Sobel, D. (1987) *The Healing Brain: Breakthrough Discoveries about How the Brain Keeps Us Healthy*, New York: Touchstone.

Ornstein, R. and Swencionis, C. (eds) (1990) *The Healing Brain – A Scientific Reader*, New York: The Guilford Press.

Orth-Gomér, K. and Undén, A. (1990) "Type A behavior, social support, and coronary risk: interaction and significance for mortality in cardiac patients", *Psychosomatic Medicine*, **52**: 59–72.

Orth-Gomér, K., Wamala, S.P., Horsten, M., Schenck-Gustafsson, K., Schneiderman, N. and Mittleman, M.A. (2001) "Marital stress worsens prognosis in women with coronary heart disease: the Stockholm Female Coronary Risk Study", *Journal of the American Medical Association*, **284**, 23: 3008–3014.

Papakostas, Y.G. and Daras, M.D. (2001) "Placebos, placebo effect, and the response to the healing situation: the evolution of a concept", *Epilepsia*, **42**, 12: 1614–1625.

Pei, M. (1962) *The Families of Words*, New York: Saint Martin's Press.

Pennebaker, J., Barger, S. and Tiebout, J. (1989) "Disclosure of traumas and health among holocaust survivors", *Psychomatic Medicine*, **51**: 577–589.

Pennebaker, J., Kiecolt-Glaser, J. and Glaser, R. (1988) "Disclosure of traumas and immune function. Implications for psychotherapy", *Journal of Consulting Clinical Psychology*, **56**: 239–245.

Pennebaker, J. and O'Heeron, R. (1984) "Confiding in others and illness among spouses of suicide and accidental death victims", *Journal of Abnormal Psychology*, **93**: 473–476.

Pennebaker, J. and Susman, J. (1988) "Disclosure of traumas and psychosomatic processes", *Social Science Medicine*, **26**: 327–332.

Penninx, B.W., Guralnik, J.M., Pahor, M., Ferrucci, L., Cerhan, J.R., Wallace, R.B. and Havlik, R.J. (1998) "Chronically depressed mood and cancer risk in older persons", *Journal of the National Cancer Institute*, **90**, 24: 1888–1893.

Persky, V., Kempthorne-Rawson, J. and Shekelle, R. (1987) "Personality and risk of cancer: 20-year follow-up of the Western Electric Study", *Psychosomatic Medicine*, **49**: 435–449.

Plato (380 BCE) *Charmides, or Temperance* (transl. B. Jowett). http://classics.mit.edu/Plato/charmides.html. Accessed 7 January 2004.

Pope, M. and Smith, T. (1991) "Cortisol excretion in high and low cynically hostile men", *Psychosomatic Medicine*, **53**: 386–392.

Ramirez, A., Craig, T. and Watson, J. (1989) "Stress and relapse of breast cancer", *British Medical Journal*, **298**: 291–293.

Ramos, D.G. (1990) *A Psique do Coração* (The Psyche of the Heart), São Paulo: Editora Cultrix.

Reich, W. (1954/1955) *Analisis del Caracter*, Buenos Aires: Editorial Paidos.

Reichel-Dolmatoff, G. (1971) *Amazonian Cosmos. The Sexual Religious Symbolism of the Tukano Indians*, Chicago: The University of Chicago Press.

Reisine, S., Fifield, J. and Winkelman, D.K. (1998) "Employment patterns and their effect on health outcomes among women with rheumatoid arthritis followed for 7 years", *Journal of Rheumatology*, **25**, 10: 1908–1916.

Rice, D. (1979) "No lung cancer in schizophrenics?", *British Journal of Psychiatry*, **134**: 128.

Rosenkrantz, B.G. (1985) "The search for professional order in 19th century American medicine", in J.W. Leavitt and R. Numbers (eds), *Sickness and Health in America*, Madison, WI: University of Wisconsin Press.

Rossi, E.L. (1986) *The Psychobiology of Mind–Body Healing*, New York: W.W. Norton.

Russek, L., King, S., Russek, S. and Russek, H. (1990) "The Harvard mastery of stress study 35-year follow-up: prognostic significance of patterns of psychophysiological arousal and adaptation", *Psychosomatic Medicine*, **52**: 271–285.

Sandner, D.F. (1986) *The Subjective Body in Clinical Practice*, Wilmette, IL: Chiron, pp. 1–17.

Santos, F. and Otelo, C. (1992) "Histeria, Hipocondria e Fenômeno Psicossomático", in J. Mello Filho *et al.*, *Psicossomática Hoje*, Porto Alegre, Brazil: Editora Artes Médicas Sul.

Schleifer, S., Keller, S., Camarino, E., Thornton, J. and Stein, M. (1983) "Suppression of lymphocyte stimulation following bereavement", *Journal of the American Medical Association*, **250**: 374–377.

Selye, H. (1956) *The Stress of Life*, New York: McGraw-Hill.

Sephton, S. and Spiegel, D. (2003) "Circadian disruption in cancer: a neuroendocrine-immune pathway from stress to disease?", *Brain, Behavior, and Immunity*, **17**, 5: 321–328.

Shaffer, J.W., Graves, P.L., Swank, R.T. and Pearson, T.A. (1987) "Clustering of personality traits in youth and the subsequent development of cancer among physicians", *Journal of Behavioral Medicine*, **10**, 5: 441–447.

Shapiro, A.K. (1960) "A contribution to a history of the placebo effect", *Behavioral Science*, **5**: 109–135.

Shapiro, A.K. (1964) "Factors contributing to the placebo effect", *American Journal of Psychotherapy*, **73**, suppl.: 73–88.

Shapiro, A.K. and Morris, L.A. (1978) "The placebo effect in medical and psychological therapies", in S.L. Garfield and A.E. Bergin (eds), *Handbook of Psychotherapy and Behavior Change*, New York: Wiley.

Sharpe, L., Sensky, T., Timberlake, N., Ryan, B. and Allard, S. (2003) "Long-term efficacy of a cognitive behavioural treatment from a randomized controlled trial for patients recently diagnosed with rheumatoid arthritis", *Rheumatology (Oxford)*, **42**, 3: 435–441.

Sharpe, L., Sensky, T., Timberlake, N., Ryan, B., Brewin, C.R. and Allard, S. (2001) "A blind, randomized, controlled trial of cognitive–behavioural intervention for patients with recent onset rheumatoid arthritis: preventing psychological and physical morbidity", *Pain*, **89**, 2–3: 275–283.

Shekelle, R.B., Raynor, W.J. Jr, Ostfeld, A.M., Garron, D.C., Bieliauskas, L.A., Liu, S.C., Maliza, C. and Paul, O. (1981) "Psychological depression and 17-year risk of death from cancer", *Psychosomatic Medicine*, **43**, 2: 117–125.

Sidoli, M. (2000) *When the Body Speaks*, London: Routledge.

Siegman, A., Dembroski, T. and Ringel, N. (1987) "Components of hostility and the severity of coronary artery disease", *Psychosomatic Medicine*, 51: 514–522.

Siegman, A.W., Townsend, S.T., Civelek, A.C. and Blumenthal, R.S. (2000) "Antagonistic behavior, dominance, hostility, and coronary heart disease", *Psychosomatic Medicine*, **62**, 2: 248–257.

Sifneos, P. and Nehemiah, C. (1970) *Affect and Fantasy in Modern Trends in Psychosomatic Medicine*, vol. 2, London: Butterworth.

Simms, B. (1980) *Mind and Madness in Ancient Greece*, Ithaca, NY: Cornell University Press.

Sirois, B.C. and Burg, M.M. (2003) "Negative emotion and coronary heart disease. A review", *Behavior modification*, **27**, 1: 83–102.

Smuts, J.C. (1926) *Holism and Evolution*, New York: Macmillan.

Sobel, D.S. (1990) "The placebo effect: using the body's own healing mechanisms", in R. Ornstein and C. Swencionis (eds), *The Healing Brain*, New York: The Guilford Press.

Solié, P. (1976) *Médicines iniciatiques*, Paris: Epi S.A. Editeurs.

Solié, P. (1990) *Psychologie analytique et médicine psychosomatique*, Paris: Les Editions S. Veyrat.

Solomon, G. (1981) "Emotional and personality factors in the onset and course of autoimmune disease, particularly rheumatoid arthritis", in A. Adler (ed.), *Psychoneuroimmunology*, San Diego: Academic Press.

Solomon, G. (1990a) "Emotions, stress, and immunity", in R. Ornstein and C. Swencionis (eds), *The Healing Brain*, New York: The Guilford Press.

Solomon, G. (1990b) "The emerging field of psychoneuroimmunology, with a special note on AIDS", in R. Ornstein and C. Swencionis (eds) *The Healing Brain*, New York: The Guilford Press.

Spiegel, D. (1996) "Cancer and depression", *The British Journal of Psychiatry*, 30 suppl.: 109–116.

Spiegel, D. and Giese-Davis, J. (2003) "Depression and cancer: mechanisms and disease progression", *Biological Psychiatry*, **54**, 3: 269–282.

Straus, J.L. and von Ammon Cavanaugh, S. (1996) "Placebo effects. Issues for clinical practice in psychiatry and medicine", *Psychosomatics*, **37**, 4: 315–326.

Strik, J.J., Denollet, J., Lousberg, R. and Honig, A. (2003) "Comparing symptoms of depression and anxiety as predictors of cardiac events and increased healthcare consumption after myocardial infarction", *Journal of the American College of Cardiology*, **42**, 10: 1801–1807.

Suarez, E. and Williams, R. (1990) "Dimensions of hostility and reactivity", *Psychosomatic Medicine*, **52**: 558–570.

Symmons, D., Mathers, C. and Pfleger, B. (2000) "The global burden of rheumatoid arthritis in the year 2000", Geneva: World Health Organization. Available online at www3.who.int.

Temoshok, L. (1985) "Biopsychological studies on cutaneous malignant melanoma: psychosocial factors associated with prognostic indicators, progression, psychophysiology, and tumor–host response", *Social Science Medicine*, **20**: 833–840.

Temoshok, L. and Dreher, H. (1992) *The Type C Connection*, New York: Random House.

Temoshok, L., Heller, B. and Sagebiel, R. (1985) "The relationship of psychosocial factors to prognostic indicators in cutaneous malignant melanoma", *Journal of Psychosomatic Research*, **929**: 139–153.

Tijhuis, M.A., Elshout, J.R., Feskens, E.J., Janssen, M. and Kromhout, D. (2000) "Prospective investigation of emotional control and cancer risk in men (the Zutphen Elderly Study) (The Netherlands)", *Cancer Causes & Control*, **11**, 7: 589–595.

Turner, J.A., Deyo, R.A., Loeser, J.D., Von Korff, M. and Fordyce, W.E. (1994) "The importance of placebo effects in pain treatment and research", *Journal of the American Medical Association*, **271**, 20: 1609–1614.

UK Gabapentin Study Group (1990) "Gabapentin in partial epilepsy", *Lancet*, **335**: 1114–1117.

Ulmer, D. and Friedman, M. (1984) *Treating Type A Behavior and Your Heart*, New York: Knopf.

Van Egeren, L. and Sparrow, A. (1990) "Ambulatory monitoring to assess real-life cardiovascular reactivity in type A and type B subjects", *Psychosomatic Medicine*, **52**: 297–306.

Wamala, S.P., Lynch, J. and Kaplan, G.A. (2001) "Women's exposure to early and later life socio-economic disadvantage and coronary heart disease risk: the Stockholm Female Coronary Risk Study", *International Journal of Epidemiology*, **30**, 2: 275–284.

Wamala, S.P., Mittleman, M.A., Horsten, M., Schenck-Gustafsson, K. and Orth-Gomer, K. (2000) "Job stress and the occupational gradient in coronary heart disease risk in women. The Stockholm Female Coronary Risk Study", *Journal of Psychosomatic Research*, **51**, 4: 481–489.

Warner, J.H. (1986) *The Therapeutic Perspective*, Cambridge, MA: Harvard University Press.

Weil, P. (1990) *Holística: uma nova visão e abordagem do real*, São Paulo: Editora Palas Athena.

Williams, R., Suarez, E., Kuhn, C., Zimmerman, E.A. and Schanberg, S. (1991) "Biobehavioral basis of coronary-prone behavior in middle-aged men", *Psychosomatic Medicine*, **53**: 517–527.

Williams, S.A., Kasl, S.V., Heiat, A., Abramson, J.L., Krumholz, H.M. and Vaccarino, V. (2002) "Depression and risk of heart failure among the elderly: a prospective community-based study", *Psychosomatic Medicine*, **64**, 1: 6–12.

Wilson, M. (1980) "Body and mind from the cartesian point of view", in R.W. Rieber, *Body and Mind. Past, Present and Future*, New York: Academic Press.

Wolf, S. (1950) "Effects of suggestion and conditioning on the action of chemical agents in human subjects: the pharmacology of placebos", *Journal of Clinical Investigation*, **29**: 100–109.

Wulsin, L.R. and Singal, B.M. (2003) "Do depressive symptoms increase the risk for the onset of coronary disease? A systematic quantitative review", *Psychosomatic Medicine*, **65**, 2: 201–210.

Zautra, A.J., Hamilton, N.A., Potter, P. and Smith, B. (1999) "Field research on the relationship between stress and disease activity in rheumatoid arthritis", *Annals of the New York Academy of Sciences*, **876**: 397–412.

Zautra, A.J. and Smith, B.W. (2001) "Depression and reactivity to stress in older women with rheumatoid arthritis and osteoarthritis", *Psychosomatic Medicine*, **63**, 4: 687–696.

Ziegler, A.J. (1983) *Archetypal Medicine*, Dallas: Spring Publications.

Zonderman, A., Costa, P. and McCrae, R. (1989) "Depression as a risk for cancer morbidity and mortality in a nationally representative sample", *Journal of the American Medical Association*, **262**: 1191–1195.

Zumoff, B., Rosenfeld, R.S., Friedman, M., Byers, S.O., Rosenman, R.H. and Hellman, L. (1984) "Elevated daytime urinary excretion of testosterone glucuronide in men with the type A behavior pattern", *Psychosomatic Medicine*, **46**, 3: 223–225.

Index

Printed and bound by CPI Group (UK) Ltd, Croydon, CR0 4YY

23/10/2024

01777672-0003